101 AMAZING USES for ESSENTIAL OILS

FAMILIUS

FOR MY CRONIES WHo KEEP ME LAUGHING

Published by Familius LLC, www.familius.com

Familius books are available at special discounts for bulk purchases, whether for sales promotions or for family or corporate use. For more information, contact Familius Sales at 559-876-2170 or email orders@familius.com.

DISCLAIMER: The material in this book is for informational purposes only. It is not intended to be a substitute for professional medical advice, diagnosis, or treatment. Always seek the advice of your physician or other qualified healthcare provider with any questions you may have regarding a medical condition or treatment. Never disregard professional medical advice or delay in seeking it because of something you have read in this book.

Library of Congress Cataloging-in-Publication Data
2017933385

Print ISBN 9781945547164
Ebook ISBN 9781945547584

Printed in the United States of America

Edited by Lindsay Sandberg
Cover design by David Miles
Book design by Brooke Jorden and David Miles

10 9 8 7 6 5 4 3 2 1

First Edition

101 AMAZING USES for ESSENTIAL OILS

REDUCE STRESS, BOOST MEMORY, REPEL MOSQUITOES, AND 98 MORE!

Susan Branson

CONTENTS

INTRODUCTION

WHAT SMELLS SO GOOD?

The fresh scent of lemons, the soothing aroma of lavender, or the mystical fragrance of frankincense can conjure feelings of happiness, serenity, or clarity. Essential oil qualities stretch far beyond their beautiful scent and can invoke physiological changes in the both the mind and body. When inhaled, smell receptors in the nose send messages along the olfactory nerve to the part of the brain responsible for emotions and behavior. This part is also connected to other parts of the brain that control breathing, blood pressure, stress, memory, and hormones.[1] When ingested or applied topically, essential oils are small enough to penetrate the skin or other tissues within twenty minutes[2] and even cross the blood-brain barrier. The composition of each oil is unique to its source and can even vary widely within genera. Most oils are made up primarily of terpenes, which impart the particular aroma of the oil and give the plant its antimicrobial defenses. These properties, along with their antioxidant, anti-inflammatory, and pain-relieving abilities, are delivered to the individual using the oil. Essential oils do not contain vitamins, minerals, hormones, or nutrients.

These oils are volatile liquids produced from steam or hydrodistillation of plant leaves, stems, bark, flowers, seeds, or roots. The only oils produced differently are citrus oils, which are cold pressed from the citrus peels. It takes a lot of plant material to produce a small amount of oil and is the reason why pure essential oils can be quite expensive. Four thousand pounds of roses are needed to get one pound of oil; other plants don't need quite such high amounts of raw material. A pound of lavender oil can be produced from 220 pounds of lavender flowers. Essential oils are very concentrated, so a little goes a long way.

....

FROM MUMMIFICATION TO AROMATHERAPY, ESSENTIAL OIL USE THROUGHOUT HISTORY.

Long ago, our ancestors burned locally grown aromatic woods and herbs to smoke out evil spirits thought to be responsible for causing illness. As the years went on and man became more intellectually adventurous and innovative, civilizations began to use aromatic plants in healing, spiritual practice, and beauty treatments. While credit is commonly given to the Egyptians for beginning this tradition as long ago as five thousand years, similar uses of plant essences in both India and China were found around the same time.

The Egyptians burned incense from aromatic plants in religious ceremonies to help carry messages to their deities. It was the temple priests who prepared plant oils for religious and medicinal purposes, and they were so highly prized and expensive that some cost as much as precious metals and gems. One of the most famous uses of aromatic plant oils by the Egyptians was in the mummification process. Embalmers used cinnamon, myrrh, frankincense, juniper berry, and cedarwood to prepare the bodies for burial and the afterlife. During their earthly lives, oil use was widespread. Egyptians anointed their bodies with oils after bathing to soothe, condition, and perfume the skin. Cleopatra, known for her charm and allure, is said to have used them extensively in her beauty treatments. So enamored were they with the enticing scents the oils imparted that they became expert perfumers and were renowned for the quality and diversity of their perfumes. After his victorious defeat of Egypt, Julius Caesar returned to Rome with the highly prized Egyptian perfumes and tossed full bottles into the Roman crowds as a celebration.

The Yellow Emperor of China wrote a book on internal medicine over 4500 years ago that includes the uses of some aromatic oils. It is still in use as a reference today. A thousand years later, India followed suit and published their most sacred texts, the Vedas; among other things, this book documents over seven hundred substances, including sandalwood, myrrh, cinnamon, and ginger. They were used in religious ceremonies and the healing arts.

Trade with the Egyptians brought aromatic oils to the European continent. The Greek physician Hippocrates, known as the "Father of Medicine," studied and documented the effects of over three hundred plants and so strongly believed in their therapeutic value that he chose them to treat wounded soldiers and to combat the plague in Athens. The Romans were heavily influenced by the Greeks and adopted the use of plant oils not only in healthcare but for everyday use. They used them extravagantly for frequent massages and sprinkled them in warm baths and over their beds, clothes, and hair. The Greek physician Pedanius Dioscorides chose to administer to Roman soldiers during the first century so he could march with Roman armies and study the therapeutic effects of plants he discovered along the way. His writings were published in an impressive five-volume work with over six hundred plant-based remedies using peppermint, thyme, myrrh, lavender, ginger, dill, and juniper, among many others. Carrying on the work of these influential physicians was Claudius Galen, who successfully treated Roman gladiators with herbs and wrote extensively about the medicinal uses of plants.

Up until about a thousand years ago, oils from plants were likely extracted by solvents or pressing. It was the Persians who were the first to actually distill oils. It is this process that is still used today.

Crusaders returning home from the Holy Wars brought new perfumes, aromatics, rose water, and healing remedies to Western Europe. People decorated their homes with herbs and washed their hands in rose water, if they could afford it. After Europe plunged into the Dark Ages, much of the progress on plant oils was halted and the knowledge discarded. Medicine became governed by the Catholic Church, who decreed bathing was sinful and that all disease was a punishment from God. Plant oils were still used for their pleasing aromas and to mask the scent of filth and decay.

Despite the threat of persecution, some monks secretly tended to the sick and dying in their monasteries using herbal medicine. If they or others were found using herbs and oils, they were accused of practicing witchcraft and were either outcast or executed. By the Renaissance period, however, the use of essential oils was once again on the rise, and by the 1800s, most of Western European physicians commonly prescribed oils to combat illness. René-Maurice Gattefossé, a French chemist, coined the term *aromathérapie* to describe the use of essential oils in healing treatments, and he later wrote a book by the same name. By happenstance, Gattefossé was unfortunate enough to find out firsthand the beneficial effects of lavender in healing. He burned his hands in an accidental lab explosion. Thinking quickly, he coated his hands in lavender oil. His pain and swelling were immediately reduced, and the burned skin tissue healed quickly and without scarring.

A colleague of Gattefossé named Jean Valnet used thyme, clove, lemon, and chamomile essential oils with great success in treating wounded soldiers during the Indochina War. He wrote a book in 1964 that was later translated into *The Practice of Aromatherapy.*

Today, many doctors in Europe commonly prescribe essential oils for specific health conditions, and in North America, more and more people are complementing conventional treatments with visits to naturopaths, aromatherapists, homeopaths, chiropractors, and acupuncturists who use essential oils as part of their practices. Researchers continue the work of earlier investigators by carrying out scientifically designed research protocols in an attempt to determine the chemical constituents and physiological activity by which these remarkable oils help us heal, inside and out.

WHAT'S THE BEST WAY TO STORE ESSENTIAL OILS?

Essential oils are volatile, meaning they evaporate if left exposed to the air. Always make sure the cap is tightly screwed on the bottle to prevent the oil from disappearing before you've had a chance to use it all. Prolonged heat exposure or repeated heating and cooling also speeds up the process of evaporation. Keep your oils away from sunlight and store in a dark place.

Never put them near candles, fires, or other flames. These oils are flammable. Essential oils are not meant to be heated by candles; this is a job for diluted scents in a carrier oil. The bottles essential oils are stored in should be darkly colored and made of glass. Pure essential oils can eat into plastic, so never decant these oils into plastic bottles. Today, glass bottles can most often be found in dark amber, brown, green, and blue. Amber and brown are the most effective in keeping damaging ultraviolet rays of the sun out to prevent free radical formation. Green and blue are less effective.[3] Free radicals degrade the quality of the oil, changing its chemical composition and making it less aromatic and therapeutically effective. Oxygenation does this as well.

When oils are exposed to oxygen, it reacts with some of the chemicals in the oil. All oils are prone to oxidation, but some are much more susceptible and are better stored in a fridge. Citrus essential oils contain large amounts of limonene, which oxidizes easily. Blue oils like yarrow, blue tansy, and blue chamomile are another group of oils that oxidize more easily. You'll know these oils have lost their effectiveness if they turn from a blue to a green color. Try to use these oils within nine months to a year of purchase. Tea tree, fir, and pine oils also have a relatively short lifespan and should not be stored for more than eighteen months. Most other essential oils should remain fresh for up to two years. A few, like sandalwood and patchouli, get even better with age and are known to be stable for six to ten years or more.

HOW DO I USE ESSENTIAL OILS?

Each essential oil is made up of complex biochemical compounds that impart specific benefits to the body. They are very concentrated, so it is important to remember that a little goes a long way. Follow the label recommendations for appropriate dosing to avoid toxicity. When it comes to essential oils, remember: less is more. Obtaining the benefits of essential oils can be achieved through ingesting the oils, applying them topically, or inhaling them.

Replacing spices and herbs with essential oils or adding a few drops to water, smoothies, or yogurt are a few ways to ingest oils. By this method, essential oils enter the blood via the gastrointestinal tract where they are readily transported to the organs of the body, including the brain, and act at the cellular level. There is controversy surrounding the safety of consuming oils due to their highly concentrated nature. Toxicity is a real concern. To be safe, consult a health professional beforehand or consider using fresh or dried herbs, spices, teas, or tinctures to get the benefit of the plant's essence through this method.

Topical application to the skin is an effective and safe way to use essential oils. Apply to the forehead, soles of the feet, neck, chest, arms, or legs or add a few drops to a warm bath. Avoid direct application to the eyes and injured and inflamed skin. Essential oils are lipid soluble and will penetrate the skin to provide a localized benefit. Massage to the area will increase blood absorption and carry the oils throughout the body. Most essential oils should be diluted in a carrier oil like virgin coconut oil, jojoba oil, or sweet almond oil (if no nut allergies) before using on the skin. Typically, a 3 percent solution is recommended. This equates to three drops of essential oil to one teaspoon of carrier oil. Make sure to test the diluted oil on a small patch of skin before using over larger areas to make sure it doesn't irritate the skin. A few oils like lavender, tea tree, helichrysum, and chamomile are thought to be safe to use undiluted. However, these can also cause sensitivity, so it is advisable to dilute them as well.

The safest method to use essential oils is through inhalation. Diffusers have become very popular over the last few years and work by dispersing the oils (in water) into the air with a cool mist. When inhaled, the oils are absorbed through the alveoli of the lungs as well as the smell receptors in the nose, which prompts the olfactory nerve to send messages to the part of the brain responsible for emotions and behavior. There is also a connection to other parts of the brain that control breathing, blood pressure, stress, memory, and hormones.[4] Breathing in the enticing aroma of essential oils can have a powerful effect on the mind and body. It is not necessary to have a diffuser for this method. Adding a few drops of oil to a spray bottle with water is an excellent way to freshen clothes, furniture, or rooms.

ARE ESSENTIAL OILS SAFE?

Unless an essential oil is being claimed as a treatment for a specific disease, they are not subject to regulation by the US Food and

Drug Administration and are generally recognized as safe. This does not mean all oils are safe under all conditions. Each oil contains its own chemical makeup, and some of these chemicals can induce adverse skin reactions, resulting in irritation, phototoxicity, and sensitization. Bitter orange, lime, lemon, lemon verbena, grapefruit, angelica root, and bergamot can cause changes in skin pigmentation and a higher risk of sunburn when exposed to ultraviolet rays. When used, stay out of the sun and tanning beds for twenty-four hours. Other oils are known dermal irritants and can cause skin redness and pain. Make sure to dilute such oils in a carrier before use and never use on inflamed or injured skin.

Exposure to some essential oils can cause allergic reactions. In these cases, the first application often results in only a slight reaction. Subsequent use, however, can induce a severe inflammatory reaction producing swollen, red, and sometimes painful skin. Because everyone reacts differently, predicting which oils will be dermal sensitizers can be difficult, but a few known ones to use with caution are aniseed, sweet basil, holy basil, West Indian basil, black pepper, Virginia cedarwood, citronella, lemongrass, Peru balsam, oregano, pine, summer and winter savory, spruce, tea tree, thyme, turmeric, and ylang-ylang.

Some contraindications with blood-thinning medications and cinnamon leaf and sweet birch essential oils exist. Such oils interact with heart medications and cause the blood to become too thin, leading to internal bleeding. Those taking several medications need to be wary of sweet birch, cinnamon leaf, dill seed, sweet fennel, myrtle, nutmeg tarragon, lemon balm, winter savory, and summer savory. Silver fir and pine should be avoided in people with respiratory problems; juniper berry in those with kidney conditions; sage, thyme, rosemary, and hyssop in people with high blood pressure; sage in those suffering from seizures; and valerian, if taking antidepressants.

When using oils on babies and toddlers, use sparingly. All that is needed is 1 to 3 drops in 2 tablespoons of carrier oil. The younger the infant, the more diluted the essential oil should be. In children three years of age and older, dilute 5 to 8 drops of essential oil in 2 tablespoons of carrier oil. Be careful of the oils chosen. Some should never be used for children. Peppermint contains menthol, which can stop breathing and cause jaundice in some babies.[5] Pregnant women may want to avoid the use of oils during the first few months of pregnancy. The chemical components and their metabolites can cross into the placenta and be delivered to the fetus. Depending on the concentration of the compounds and sensitivity of the fetus, a devastating toxic effect may result. That being said, there are no recorded cases of fetal developmental complications from the topical or inhaled use of essential oils under recommended dosages. During the later stages of pregnancy, these oils can be very beneficial to ease discomfort. Some oils should not be used at any time during pregnancy because they can affect hormones, can bring on contractions, or contain chemicals that are neurotoxic or teratogenic.

Always know the potential effects of each oil before using them and begin with small exposure times and concentrations to determine any sensitivities. When used properly, essential oils can be tremendously helpful.

CHAPTER 1

RESCUING PHYSICAL HEALTH

HEALTH

WELL-BEING

BEAUTY

HOME

1. ABDOMINAL PAIN

The abdomen is the part of the body between the ribcage and hips. Pain may begin in any part of the abdomen and stay localized to one spot or radiate in any number of directions. Some report sharp, stabbing pains that come and go or consistent dull aches or cramps. The pain can be acute, lasting for only a short while, or chronic, bringing discomfort for extended periods. The causes of abdominal pain are wide reaching and include indigestion, gas, constipation, food allergies, ulcers, gastrointestinal reflux, irritable bowel syndrome, or Crohn's disease. Sometimes, the pain goes away on its own, as in the case of gas, but other pain needs to be examined by a doctor. Depending on the cause, treatments often include medication to reduce inflammation, alleviate pain, or eliminate infection.

Stomach pains affect everyone at one point or another and interrupt work, school, and social outings. Often, they are more inconvenient than a cause for alarm, but the discomfort can be unsettling, especially for children. To avoid taking a trip to the doctor's office, stock up on peppermint oil. Peppermint oil is used to remove gas, relax spasms, and reduce pain. A study on 120 children with abdominal pain related to gastrointestinal disorders found that supplementation with peppermint oil capsules was more effective at reducing the severity and duration of pain over another treatment commonly used for this condition, a combination probiotic/prebiotic.[6] No side effects were noted. Despite this, peppermint oil ingestion is not recommended, especially in children. In fact, never use peppermint oil on children under the age of six. Consider massaging diluted peppermint oil on the soles of the feet or directly on the abdomen, rather than consuming, to achieve relief. Other oils to use for abdominal pain include ginger, coriander seed, chamomile, clove, lavender, fennel, and sweet orange.

2. ALLERGIES

Whether it's pollen from the trees or shrimp from the market, allergic reactions can cause minor irritations that result in a stuffy nose, watery eyes, or mild headache or potentially be so severe as to threaten life. They happen when the immune system reacts to a substance, whether it's swirling through in the air, absorbed through the skin, or eaten for lunch. While these substances don't cause a problem for most people, the immune system doesn't recognize them in those with allergies. It sees them as unwelcome invaders and launches an attack against them. Specific antibodies are produced for each allergen that identify it as harmful to the body. Every time a person comes in contact with that allergen, the allergic response is activated.

There is no cure for allergies, but there are many over-the-counter and prescription drugs available to help ease symptoms. Among these are antihistamines, decongestants, and corticosteroids. They can cause drowsiness, high blood pressure, insomnia, irritability, restricted urine flow, muscle weakness, fluid retention, and weight gain. And these are just some of the side effects! Often, this seems like trading one set of symptoms for another.

Lavender oil can inhibit allergic reactions that set in suddenly from food or environmental irritants. In a concentration-dependent manner, they have been shown in rats to inhibit the release of histamine from mast cells and tumor necrosis cells in the peritoneum. Mast cells are part of the immune system that release histamine in response to allergens in the body. In an attempt to rid the body of the offending allergens, histamine promotes inflammation and mucus production, giving rise to congestion, runny noses, itchy eyes, or even anaphylaxis. Topical and intradermal application of lavender oil can prevent this.[7] Other oils commonly used to reduce the symptoms of allergies are peppermint, lemon, tea tree, helichrysum, German chamomile, and eucalyptus.

3. ARTHRITIS

Arthritis is the most common disability in the United States,[8] affecting more than fifty million people. There are many types, but the two most common are osteoarthritis and rheumatoid arthritis.

Osteoarthritis is characterized by inflammation of the joints. The joints provide the connection between bones that allow for movement. They are cushioned by cartilage that allow the joint to move smoothly and easily. This disease affects many people as they age due to natural wear and tear. Heredity plays a role, as does injury from trauma or disease. Those afflicted suffer from joints that are painful, creaky, stiff, and swollen. Their range of motion is reduced, particularly in the hands, feet, spine, hips, and knees. In osteoarthritis, the cartilage breaks down and inflammation sets in. Extra fluid is produced in the joint, resulting in swelling. Reducing the stress on the joint cartilage is recommended to alleviate some of the symptoms. This involves losing weight and avoiding certain activities. The goal of treatment is to reduce pain and inflammation to allow for more comfortable movement. Medications are taken as pills, creams, gels, and even injections into the arthritic joint. Side effects of these can include gastrointestinal distress such as stomach upset, diarrhea, or ulcers.

Rheumatoid arthritis is an autoimmune disorder in which the immune system mistakenly attacks its own body tissues. The lining of the joints become painfully swollen and can lead to bone erosion and joint deformity over time. Symptoms can spread to other non-joint tissues of the body. It's not known what causes this disease, but genetics combined with environmental triggers are suspected. This chronic disease is without a cure and is managed mostly through medications. Nonsteroidal anti-inflammatory drugs, steroids, or disease-modifying antirheumatic drugs can be prescribed to reduce pain, swelling, and joint damage. Possible side effects include digestive problems, liver and kidney damage, heart problems, thinning of bones, diabetes, weight gain, and severe lung infections.

Many essential oils like clove, oregano, rosemary, lemon, and lavender contain phenolic and other compounds that are known antioxidants. Antioxidants can stop the action of reactive oxygen species and free radicals that cause joint degradation in arthritis.[9] Other oils that contain anti-inflammatory compounds can reduce swelling and pain in the joints. Some essential oils used for their anti-inflammatory properties include frankincense, peppermint, myrrh, ginger, lavender, rosemary, and eucalyptus. Applying any of these or combinations of them in a carrier oil can reduce inflammation, ease pain, and increase mobility. The effects of a 20 percent essential oil ointment applied topically at the onset of arthritis were studied in rats with arthritis. Compared to placebo, rats treated with the essential oils developed less severe arthritic symptoms. Significant reduction in the amount of pro-inflammatory compounds that cause swelling and enzymes that decrease the amount of synovial fluid was found. Sixteen essential oils were blended in a carrier oil in this study (basil, bitter orange, black pepper, clary sage, cedarwood, clove bud, eucalyptus, foraha, fennel, ginger, helichrysum, lavender, nutmeg, pine needle, rosemary, and sage). The effects were attributed to the essential oils and not the carrier oil.[10]

4. ATHLETE'S FOOT

Wearing sandals in locker rooms and around public pools can help protect feet from a common fungal infection known as athlete's foot. This fungus is highly contagious and can be acquired by sharing shoes, walking on infected surfaces, or directly contacting the skin of an infected foot. Once contracted, the fungus grows on or just under the surface of the skin and thrives in moist, warm places. It's important to dry the feet well, particularly between the toes, to prevent fungus from growing. The fungi can also grow in shoes, so make sure to disinfect all footwear as well.

There are three types of infection. Toe web type occurs between the toes, causing the skin to become itchy, scaly, dry, and cracked. Moccasin type is characterized by a sore foot, followed by thickened skin on the heel or along the bottom of the foot. Vesicular athlete's foot develops as blisters under the skin. Mild infections can be treated with antifungal lotions, but more severe infections may require prescription antifungal topical medications or pills.

Tea tree oil can help alleviate the symptoms of athlete's foot by destroying the fungi that colonizes the skin and causes inflammation. Patients with athlete's foot were randomized into a double-blind study and received one of two dilutions of tea tree oil or placebo. Over the next four weeks, participants applied the solutions topically twice a day. The more highly concentrated tea tree oil group showed cure rates of more than double the patients in the placebo group. Tea tree oil is not alone in its antifungal properties. Aegle, citronella, geranium, peppermint, eucalyptus, lemongrass, orange, palmarosa, and patchouli were tested against eleven fungi and found to inhibit growth of them all.[11] Next time a case of athlete's foot takes hold, mix any of these oils in a carrier oil like grapeseed oil, apricot kernel oil, or argan oil and massage into the skin of the foot twice a day.

5. BLADDER CANCER

The balloon-shaped, hollow organ in the pelvis that stores urine after it has left the kidneys is called the bladder. It has flexible, muscular walls that contract to send urine out of the body. The cells lining these walls can mutate and grow uncontrollably, eventually forming a tumor. If left unchecked, this cancer can spread to lymph nodes or other parts of the body. Most cases are caught in the early stages and are suspected when there is blood in the urine accompanied by back or pelvic pain. Frequent and painful urination may also occur. Depending on how advanced the cancer is, surgery is often indicated to remove the tumor. Sometimes, sections or the entire bladder are removed at the same time. Chemotherapy drugs and radiation therapy to kill the cancer cells may be administered before or after surgery.

Frankincense oil shows promise in fighting bladder cancer cells. This oil was tested for its activity on human bladder cancer and normal cells. In the cancer cells, frankincense oil activated genes that induced cell death. Normal cells were unaffected.[12] Along with doctor-recommended conventional treatment, diluted frankincense can be massaged into the pelvic region of the skin or inhaled by diffuser.

Adding lavender into the mix will help relieve fatigue. Twenty terminally ill cancer patients suffering from high levels of fatigue during advanced stages of their disease were given lavender oil in aromatherapy, followed by a three-minute lavender footbath and lavender reflexology treatments. All patients improved their physical and cognitive fatigue scores.[13]

6. CANDIDIASIS

Candidiasis is a fungal infection caused by the yeast-like *Candida* fungus. There are over twenty species of *Candida* that can infect humans, but *Candida albicans* is the most common. These yeasts normally live on the skin and mucous membranes in people and are generally harmless. If conditions in the body shift to create an environment favorable to *Candida* overgrowth, infections of the mouth, vagina, urinary tract, skin, or stomach can set in. Most causes of *Candida* overgrowth result from certain drugs, pregnancy, bacterial infections, excess weight, or an overburdened immune system. Vaginal yeast infections, white lesions on the tongue or inner cheek, painful cracks in the skin at the corners of the mouth, or crusted skin rashes around the fingers, toes, and groin are symptoms of candidiasis. Antifungal drugs are commonly prescribed for up to two weeks.

Reducing sugar and yeast products in the diet and taking probiotics are popular alternative therapies to getting rid of candidiasis. Essential oils can be used alongside these practices. Lavender oil was tested against fifty-one strains of *Candida albicans* in a laboratory setting. It effectively inhibited fungal growth and reduced the spread of infection.[14] Eugenol, found in clove, geranium, oregano, nutmeg, and cinnamon oil, inhibited thirty-one strains of *Candida albicans*.[15] Manuka, helichrysum, sweet marjoram, patchouli, peppermint, lemongrass, and tea tree are oils also used for antifungal purposes. They may work by decreasing lipid content and altering the outer surface of the yeast cells or by interfering with the yeast's enzymatic reactions. Candidiasis is very common, so consider using essential oils as either a preventative measure or as a safe alternative to antifungal drugs.

7. CAVITIES

The mouth is full of bacteria. Some are helpful, and others are harmful. The harmful bacteria form a sticky, colorless substance that adheres to the teeth and gum line. This is called plaque. Plaque loves to feed on sugars and starches, so nearly every meal provides plaque with fuel for growth. As the bacteria in the plaque feed on the sugars, they produce acids. These acids demineralize the tooth surface by extracting calcium and phosphate from the enamel.

Saliva tries to neutralize the acids and provide the missing minerals so that the tooth enamel can remineralize. When demineralization happens faster than remineralization, the tooth begins to decay, creating holes or cavities. Cavities are a major oral health concern and affect up to 90 percent of schoolchildren and the majority of adults. The only treatment for cavities is to drill out the decay and fill the hole with composite resins, porcelain, or amalgams.

Once a cavity has begun, the process cannot be reversed. The best course of action is to prevent tooth decay before it starts. A good oral hygiene routine is essential and should involve flossing and brushing twice daily. Reducing sugar consumption can also help to lower acid output from bacteria that cause enamel erosion. As an added measure, essential oil can be used to inhibit bacterial growth in the mouth. Peppermint and sage oils are potent in reducing oral bacteria[16] and can be used in a mouthwash in the morning and evening to lower cavity-inducing bacterial counts and protect the teeth from acid erosion. Add 3 drops of peppermint oil in 1 teaspoon of virgin coconut oil and swish around the mouth for several minutes. Spit out in the garbage and brush your teeth as normal.

8. COLDS AND FLU

Common colds and seasonal flu are respiratory illnesses caused by different viruses. They are highly contagious, and a person can become infected by touching a surface such as a doorknob, stair railing, or bathroom faucet. If the virus gets on the hands and the person then touches their mouth or nose, the virus nestles into the mucosal lining there. Breathing in air near someone who is coughing or sneezing while they are sick with a cold or the flu is another surefire way of getting the virus into the system. There are many different viruses that cause colds and flus. Unless the body has fought the exact virus before, it won't have the right antibodies ready to fight it when it enters the body. The immune system begins an attack against the new virus, and the dreaded symptoms set in. A sore throat, runny or stuffy nose, sneezing, and cough are the hallmarks of a cold. If these symptoms are accompanied by a fever, fatigue, and muscle aches, it is more likely to be the flu. There is no shortage of over-the-counter cold and flu medications, and they are available for every possible symptom. Take a walk down the pharmacy aisle to see antihistamines, decongestants, nasal sprays, cough suppressants, and throat lozenges.

Essential oils have been used as effective home remedies for centuries to combat the unpleasant and uncomfortable symptoms of cold and flu. A blend of wild orange, clove, cinnamon, eucalyptus, and rosemary oils was shown to inhibit viral proliferation of the influenza virus PK8 in a laboratory setting.[17] Eucalyptus and pine oils can open the airways, help clear the sinuses, and relieve a sore throat. Thyme, frankincense, tea tree, and rosemary help thin mucus and reduce chest and nasal congestion. Greek sage, sweet fennel, lemon, clove, and lavender essential oils are others commonly used in various combinations to reduce the symptoms and shorten the duration of colds and flu. Many of these oils have antimicrobial compounds and are thought to work by lowering the viral load or by boosting the immune system so the body can better fight the invading pathogens. They can be used as a preventative or in the treatment of existing infections.

Massage diluted lavender and frankincense oils onto the chest, the temples, or the back of the neck several times a day, or add eucalyptus, thyme, tea tree, and lemon oils to a warm bath and relax for twenty minutes.

9. COLD SORES

Cold sores, or fever blisters, are herpes simplex viral infections that affect the skin around the mouth. Fluid-filled sores develop in and around the lips that eventually break, leaking a clear liquid. A crust then forms. Cold sores tend to group in clusters, are red, swollen, and sore, and can be accompanied by fever and swollen neck glands. Some cold sores last only a few days, while others take weeks to go away. The herpes simplex virus is contagious, and touching the area or sharing utensils, toothbrushes, or razors can spread the infection. The virus gets into the skin though any scratch or tiny cut, so if an outbreak is underway, don't kiss anyone goodnight or share a glass of wine! Once the virus is contracted, it will always be there. It is not precisely known why an outbreak occurs, but stress and a depressed immune system are thought to be triggers. Treating with antiviral creams, ointments, or pills can reduce symptoms but usually get rid of the cold sores only one or two days quicker than without treatment.

An outbreak of cold sores is not only painful but can be embarrassing for some individuals. The initial tingling sensation associated with an impending outbreak can have a person reaching for medication or send them into hiding until the cold sores have cleared up.

Nine essential oils were found to inhibit the growth of herpes simplex virus type 1, the type that causes cold sores. One percent solutions of each oil were incubated with the herpes viruses and then added to cell cultures, where they suppressed the viruses by inactivating their genetic material. The most effective oil was lemongrass, which was able to completely inhibit growth at concentrations as low as 0.1 percent. The other effective oils were tea tree, peppermint, marjoram, eucalyptus, ravensara, lavender, lemon, and rosemary.[18] At the first sign of an outbreak, apply a 1 percent solution (one drop of essential oil in 1 teaspoon of carrier oil), using any of the above oils, to the affected area of the mouth several times a day to stop the virus from replicating and spreading.

10. CONSTIPATION

Constipation is infrequent bowel movements or difficulty in passing stools. It is very common and can be occasional or chronic. Occasional constipation is short term, while chronic constipation is having less than three bowel movements a week for at least three months. It is a result of stools moving too slowly through the digestive tract, causing them to become hard and dry. They are difficult to pass, and a feeling of not being able to empty the rectum is reported. Increasing fiber intake, fluids, and exercise are known to help increase gastric motility. If that doesn't work, laxatives and other medications to draw water into the intestines are suggested. Side effects of these drugs include bloating, gas, diarrhea, nausea, vomiting, and rectal pain.

Constipation can be very distressing and impact quality of life. Aromatherapy massage with essential oils has been shown to relieve constipation. Elderly patients suffering from constipation received abdominal massage with rosemary, peppermint, and lemon essential oils for ten days. Severity of the condition decreased and the number of bowel movements increased, compared to the patients in the control group who received a placebo abdominal massage with no essential oils.[19] Sweet marjoram, patchouli, sweet fennel, and ginger are some other essential oils that can be used to stimulate bowel movements. Add 1 drop of sweet marjoram oil and 2 drops of peppermint oil to 1 teaspoon of sweet almond oil and massage over the abdomen in a clockwise direction. Do this several times a day until no longer needed.

11. CUTS AND SCRAPES

Wounding the skin is a very common occurrence and happens to everyone. Whether it's slicing the tip of the finger while dicing carrots or slipping on gravel and scraping a knee, any cuts or scrapes tear the skin tissue and, often, cause bleeding. If the wound is deep, bleeds heavily, or has an object embedded in it, seek medical attention. If it's minor, however, it can be addressed at home. Wash your hands with soap and water. Clean the cut or scrape by pouring cool, clean water over it to remove dirt and debris. Then wash with soap and water. Once clean, an antibiotic ointment can be applied.

Myrrh has been used as a traditional wound healing medication for over 4000 years by royalty and commoners alike, both on the battlefield and in the home. Recent evidence confirms its effectiveness in healing injured tissue. Damaged skin in mice treated with an ointment made from myrrh essential oil healed more quickly than wounded skin in mice treated with a control ointment. New, stronger skin cells were laid down at a faster pace and closed the wound in less time.[20]

Infections by opportunistic pathogens are common in wounds that are not cleaned properly. Not only does myrrh aid in speeding up wound healing, it acts as an antimicrobial agent against bacteria and fungi. It is as effective as standard antibiotic and antifungal medications.[21] Using myrrh on wounds will speed healing and prevent infection. Lavender, tea tree, sweet marjoram, myrtle, neroli, niaouli, rose, patchouli, sandalwood, and frankincense oils are some others also used to heal cuts and other superficial wounds.

12. DEMENTIA

Dementia is a term used to describe a range of symptoms that weakens mental ability and affects daily living. Alzheimer's disease accounts for the majority of dementia cases, followed by vascular dementia, which can occur after a stroke. It is caused by damage to brain cells that prevents normal communication and functioning, resulting in impaired memory, focus, communication, reasoning, and coordination. Changes in personality are also common and can include agitation, paranoia, anxiety, depression, and hallucinations. Some cases of dementia are reversible, and others are progressive. For most, there is no cure. Symptoms can be managed through medications, but these run the risk of adverse effects like nausea, vomiting, dizziness, and diarrhea. Pet therapy, art therapy, music therapy, massage therapy, and aromatherapy are alternatives being explored to promote relaxation.

The use of aromatherapy has been found to have beneficial effects in reducing agitation in patients suffering from severe dementia. Agitated behavior in fifteen dementia patients significantly improved after 2 percent lavender oil was diffused in the psychogeriatric ward housing them,[22] while lemon balm applied topically in a lotion to the arms and faces of dementia patients over four weeks improved not only agitation but quality of life as indicated by social interaction and time involved in productive activities.[23] Peppermint, cinnamon leaf, rosemary, and black pepper oils can be used to improve memory and enhance brain health. Combine the behavior-soothing oils with the brain-enhancing oils for added beneficial effects to reduce the symptoms of dementia.

13. DIABETES

Diabetes is a disease that affects the way the body handles glucose, resulting in high levels of this sugar in the blood. There is type 1 diabetes, in which the pancreas produces little or no insulin, type 2 diabetes, in which the pancreas does produce insulin but the body doesn't use it as well as it should, and gestational diabetes, a form of high blood sugar affecting pregnant women. Some people are genetically predisposed to diabetes, but being overweight is also a risk factor. Feelings of thirst, frequent urination, fatigue, tingling or numbness in the hands or feet, and blurry vision are all signs of diabetes. Managing diabetes involves exercising, improving diet, and monitoring blood glucose levels. For many, daily insulin injections are needed.

The high incidence of diabetes makes finding a natural alternative to manage this disease very desirable. Indian bay leaf essential oil was administered to diabetic rats for twenty-eight days. Plasma insulin levels significantly increased, while blood glucose levels significantly decreased. This oil was found to be as effective as glibenclamide, a popular antidiabetic drug, used to treat type 2 diabetes.[24] Rose-scented geranium essential oil also significantly decreased blood glucose and was even more effective than gliben-clamide.[25] Cinnamon, clove, and Korean pine oils are thought to balance blood sugar levels too. These can be used along with lav-ender and lemon oils to decrease fatigue and citronella as well as ginger and grapefruit oils to boost metabolism and enhance weight loss. Taken together, combinations of these oils may be valuable in controlling blood sugar levels, reducing risk factors, and managing the effects of diabetes in humans.

14. ESCHERICHIA COLI

E. coli are bacteria that normally live in the intestines of humans and animals. Many types of *E. coli* are harmless and are important to the health of the digestive tract. Several species, however, are pathogen-ic and cause bloody diarrhea, urinary tract infections, anemia, or kidney failure. Contraction of *E. coli* can be made from contact with infected persons or animals or from consuming food or water con-taining the bacteria. *E. coli* can contaminate meat during processing and, if it is not cooked to 160 degrees Fahrenheit, can survive and in-fect the consumer. Sometimes, cows spread the bacteria to their milk as it passes through their udders. If the milk is not pasteurized, the bacteria will continue to live and pose a threat. Even raw fruits and vegetables can have *E. coli* bacteria from contact with contaminated water or persons. Three or four days after ingesting *E. coli*, food poi-soning becomes evident as symptoms develop. They usually subside on their own after about a week.

HEALTH

WELL-BEING

BEAUTY

HOME

Anyone who has been through an episode of food poisoning understands how absolutely miserable it is. Prevention is best, so be sure to cook meats to their proper temperature and wash produce to remove any offending pathogens. Essential oils are effective, natural, and safe substances that can inhibit the growth of *E. coli* on food and potentially save an outbreak of food poisoning in the household. Laboratory tests discovered the growth-suppressing action of thyme, oregano, clove, nutmeg, and black pepper essential oils on *E. coli*,[26] and oregano oil was even able to kill a multidrug-resistant strain within ten minutes.[27] Juniper and chrysanthemum oils were also shown to inhibit *E. coli* growth.[28] After purchasing produce, add a mixture of 3 drops of thyme oil, 2 drops of oregano oil, and 2 drops of juniper oil to a cup of water. Shake solution before you spray produce. Rinse produce after fifteen minutes. To increase germ-fighting power, add 1/4 cup apple cider vinegar to the bottle.

If *E. coli* has entered the system and symptoms have developed, add a few drops of peppermint oil or ginger oil to a cotton ball and inhale for several minutes. Nausea should subside.

15. EXERCISE PERFORMANCE

Aerobic exercise improves fitness by increasing heart and breathing rates for a duration of longer than a few minutes. Blood gets pumped around the body, delivering oxygen to the cells to keep the muscles working. Increasing fitness improves not only physical health but mental and emotional health as well. Regular aerobic exercise strengthens the heart, makes the muscles more efficient at consuming oxygen, and increases the number of mitochondria in the muscle cells. These increase endurance and more efficiently burn fat and carbohydrates. Running, walking, biking, and swimming are some examples of aerobic activity. It's important to work anaerobically, too. This type of exercise is short and intense. It relies on oxygen already stored in the muscles and is primarily performed to build muscle. Lifting weights or resistance training, using body weight, can do this. Weight training breaks down muscles, and during repair, there is new and larger growth of muscle tissue. It is theorized that the muscles get larger to protect the body from future stresses.

Fitness begins with being active and committing to daily activity. Increasing fitness is a goal many of us have, and there are numerous products on the market that promise to do this by improving stamina or building muscle. Some of these may work, but they often have a long list of questionable ingredients. Enhancing performance by using pure essential oils can be a safe and effective means to help reach these goals. Peppermint essential oil consumed by healthy male subjects for ten days significantly increased the amount of work, power, and duration of a treadmill-based exercise they were able to do compared to prior results.[29] Oils can be used pre- and post-workout to prepare the body for exercise and ensure recovery time is minimal. Before a workout, massage diluted ginger and rosemary oils over the muscles to warm them up and give the body a boost of energy. Afterward, take a soothing bath with lavender, eucalyptus, and sweet marjoram oils to decrease inflammation and provide relief from muscle spasms and cramps.

HEALTH

WELL-BEING

BEAUTY

HOME

16. FEVER

Fever is a temporary increase in the body's temperature. It is not an illness but a sign that something unusual is happening in the body. Mild fevers should be left untreated to allow the immune system to take care of the cause. Higher fevers are of more concern and require some intervention. Sweating, chills, fatigue, muscle weakness, and headache may accompany fevers. They are generally caused by viruses, bacteria, some medications, sunburn, inflammatory conditions, and malignant tumors. Over-the-counter medications such as aspirin and acetaminophen or prescribed antibacterial drugs are effective in reducing fever, but those come with risks. Antibiotics destroy good intestinal bacteria, causing digestive upset, overuse of acetaminophen can cause kidney and liver damage, and aspirin can cause stomach pain, unusual bleeding, and weakness.

Numerous essential oils have been used for centuries to reduce or break fevers. Holy basil has been proven to lower vaccine-induced fever in rats, having comparable effects to aspirin. No long-term effects of using holy basil were found.[30] Clove oil contains a compound called eugenol. This has been found to decrease fever in rabbits and is more effective than acetaminophen.[31] Eugenol is also found in geranium, oregano, nutmeg, and basil essential oils. Others long considered to reduce body temperature include peppermint, eucalyptus, frankincense, lavender, black cumin, sage, patchouli, lemongrass, ginger, and hyssop oils. Any of these oils can be inhaled, used topically, or sprinkled in a warm bath. Apply 3 drops of sage oil on a wet washcloth and place over the forehead, repeating three times a day. For children over six years of age, dilute 1 drop of peppermint oil in 1 teaspoon of coconut oil and dab on the bottom of the feet and back of the neck. When the fever starts to rise again, repeat.

17. FIBROMYALGIA

This disorder is characterized by widespread muscle pain and tenderness. It is thought that the brains of those with fibromyalgia process pain signals differently and amplify painful sensations. Sleep is often disrupted, fatigue constant, memory impaired, and mood altered. Symptoms can occur gradually over time or be triggered by severe stress, infection, surgery, or trauma. Those suffering from fibromyalgia can take medications for pain or antidepressants to help with sleep. As with any medication, side effects are not uncommon—nausea, rashes, upset stomach, weight gain, and sexual problems are just a few.

Essential oils can be used by fibromyalgia patients to improve their quality of life. Reduction in pain is a primary endpoint for most patients. This can be achieved by using the essential oil from *Xylopia laevigata*, a medicinal plant used in folk remedies to treat pain and inflammation. A recent study confirms its effectiveness.[32] Oral treatment with basil essential oil reduced sensitivity to pain in a mice fibromyalgia model,[33] and lemon essential oil influenced the behavior and nervous system responses to painful stimulation in rats.[34] Inhaling or applying these (diluted) essential oils on the skin can reduce debilitating pain, providing relief to the patient.

Grapefruit, sweet marjoram, and lavender oils can help relieve fatigue that often plagues fibromyalgia patients and leaves them unable to perform their daily tasks. Those that find their memory fading or concentration waning will certainly perk up after using peppermint, rosemary, lemon, and cardamom oils that can improve memory. Having more energy and less pain may be enough to lift the spirits, but clary sage, bergamot, neroli, frankincense, or rosemary oil can boost mood with their antidepressant-like effects. Using a combination of several of these oils should help alleviate the symptoms of fibromyalgia.

18. FLATULENCE

Gas can accumulate in the digestive tract. It gets there from swallowing little bits of air with our food, drink, or saliva and from the digestion of food. As gas builds up, the body needs to get rid of it, either by belching or flatulating. Everyone produces gas, and it is usually not serious. Excessive gas buildup can cause bloating, stomach cramps, and intestinal pain. To avoid excessive gas and the symptoms that come with it, a change in lifestyle and diet are usually all that are needed. Eating smaller meals more frequently, chewing thoroughly, exercising, and avoiding gas-producing foods and chewing gum are recommended.

Still, sometimes a little outside help is needed. Peppermint and clove oils relax digestive muscles, allowing gas to pass. Ginger stimulates muscle contractions of the stomach,[35] moving gas through the digestive system for expulsion. Coriander seed, cardamom, caraway seed, sweet fennel, and black pepper, among many others, all support the digestive system and can reduce stomach bloating and pain associated with excessive gas. Blend a drop each of peppermint, cardamom, and coriander seed essential oils with a teaspoon of jojoba oil and massage in a clockwise fashion over the abdominal area.

19. GASTRIC ULCERS

Ulcers are holes in the protective lining of the stomach, small intestine, and esophagus. Sores develop that may cause stomach pain, bloating, heartburn, nausea, and fatty food intolerance. Infection with *H. pylori* is thought to be the main cause. Overuse of painkillers, smoking, stress, and heavy alcohol use are other contributing factors. If *H. pylori* are present, treatment involves a course of antibiotics to kill the bacteria. Medications to neutralize, block, or reduce the production of stomach acid are often prescribed. It is imperative that the use of painkillers, smoking, and alcohol use is greatly reduced or stopped.

The essential oils of two members of the Lamiaceae family of plants have been shown to have gastroprotective effects and help heal gastric ulcers. *Hyptis martiusii*, a common flowering plant in Brazil, reduced acidity and the amount of gastric secretions in the stomachs of laboratory rats. Mucus production was increased, protecting the lining of the stomach from acid injury. New, healthy tissue regrows, and ulcer size is reduced.[36] *Thymus algeriensis*, a related plant that grows abundantly in North Africa, significantly reduced the size of gastric ulcers in study rats with a single oral dose.[37] If *H. pylori* is responsible for the development of ulcers, then eradicating them in the stomach will allow gastric tissues to heal. The essential oils of peppermint and spearmint can do just this.

They are effective in inhibiting the growth of both antibiotic-resistant and antibiotic-sensitive strains of *H. pylori*.[38] Other oils used to heal or prevent the development of ulcers are frankincense, ginger, fennel, lemongrass, and myrtle. Take 2 drops each of peppermint, ginger, and myrtle and mix in a teaspoon of argan oil. Massage over the stomach. Repeat several times a day until symptoms disappear.

20. GINGIVITIS

Gingiva is the part of the gum around the base of the teeth that becomes diseased and causes gingivitis. The gums tend to bleed easily, become puffy, and turn from pink to red. When inflamed, they begin to recede, and tooth decay sets in. Gingivitis is caused when hardened plaque, called tartar, forms below and above the gum line. Tartar is full of bacteria, and it is the bacteria that begin the infection. Plaque is formed daily on the teeth, but it can easily be removed through daily brushing and flossing. If it is left to harden into tartar, it is much harder to eliminate. This disease is common and symptoms are often mild, so most people don't know they have it. Professional teeth cleaning is needed, followed by a good oral hygiene routine at home.

In addition to regular brushing, many people use antibacterial mouthwashes to get rid of oral bacteria in the mouth responsible for plaque formation leading to gingivitis. Many of these products contain compounds like chlorhexidine, triclosan, and hydrogen peroxide, which can irritate the skin and respiratory tissue. Preservatives and flavoring agents are usually added, some of these known to disrupt hormones. Pure essential oils can safely be diluted in carrier oils and used to rinse the mouth and help keep gingivitis from developing. A double-blind clinical study tested a 10 percent pepper rosemary essential oil gel for its inhibitory effects on plaque development in the mouth. After three weeks, gingivitis was effectively controlled compared to the test group.[39] In fact, a systematic review of studies testing a variety of essential oil mouthwashes on plaque development and gingival inflammation found that these mouthwashes were as effective as commercial mouthwashes containing the commonly used antiseptic agent chlorhexidine. Cinnamon leaf, peppermint, spearmint, lemon, and clove essential oils all have antiseptic properties and can be used to combat oral bacteria and reduce the risk of gingivitis. After brushing the teeth each morning, dilute 2 drops of cinnamon leaf essential oil in a teaspoon of virgin coconut oil and swish around the mouth for thirty seconds to a minute. Spit in the garbage to prevent clogging the sink drain.

21. HEADACHES AND MIGRAINES

A headache is a pain in any part of the head and may be sharp, dull, or throbbing. It can last from under an hour to several days. Migraines are severe headaches that cause intense pain, usually on one side of the head, and are accompanied by nausea, vomiting, and sensitivity to light and sound. Migraines can come with warning signs such as blind spots in the field of vision, flashes of light, or tingling sensations on the face, arms, or legs. Migraines can be so severe that the person can't function normally and often requires rest and isolation to recover. Causes of migraines are different for everyone. Some triggers could be changes in hormone levels, food allergies, stress, some medications, sensory stimuli, or changes in the environment, like a fall in barometric pressure from an approaching storm. Regular headaches can be caused by a multitude of factors, from dehydration to too little sleep to infections. They may also be symptoms of disease. Pain-relieving medications are commonly used to deal with the symptoms. In the case of migraines, antinausea medications are also prescribed.

Peppermint essential oil can be spread across the forehead and temples to reduce the severity of tension-type headaches and provide relief. In a double-blind study, a 10 percent peppermint oil solution was used topically and found to significantly reduce pain intensity after fifteen minutes. This observation continued throughout the one-hour observation period. It was even found to be as effective as acetaminophen, and no adverse events were recorded.[40] Inhaling lavender oil for fifteen minutes has been shown to significantly reduce migraine headache severity compared to the control group, with 71 percent of participants responding positively to it.[41] Other oils to use are rosemary, Roman chamomile, lavandin, marjoram, and rosewood.

22. HOT FLASHES

When women enter their menopausal years, up to two-thirds of them experience hot flashes, the sudden onset of intense heat or warmth in the face, neck, and chest. It can be accompanied by rapid heartbeat, flushed red skin, and sweating. Each woman's experience is different. Some only have them for a short period of time, while others continue to get them throughout their lives. Whether it happens a few times a day or several times an hour, the severity of hot flashes tends to decrease over time. Around the time of menopause, a woman's reproductive hormone balance changes and the hypothalamus, which regulates the body temperature, may also be experiencing some changes. It is thought that these two may play a role in the onset of hot flashes. When the body temperature rises, the blood vessels near the surface of the skin dilate in an attempt to cool the body down. Women may opt to take hormones to prevent hot flashes if they are severe or interfere with daily life. Estrogen or a combination of estrogen and progesterone are commonly prescribed. Antidepressants and antiseizure medications are also given to reduce hot flashes. These drugs can increase the risk of breast cancer, stroke, heart disease, and blood clots. They can also cause irritability, anxiety, nausea, and fatigue. These are just some of the side effects.

For those not wanting to take hormone replacement drugs, essential oils provide an alternative that many find effective. One of the most widely used oils to reduce the frequency and severity of hot flashes is clary sage. It is thought that some of the molecules in this oil can occupy estrogen receptor sites in the body and provide support during menopause when estrogen levels are declining. Like clary sage, Roman chamomile, niaouli, geranium, and palmarosa are thought to reduce hot flashes by helping to balance hormone levels. Peppermint oil cools flushed skin and can be used with any of these oils to improve comfort. Mix 2 drops of clary sage oil with 2 drops of peppermint oil in 1 teaspoon of sweet almond oil and dab across the back of the neck and on the bottoms of the feet.

HEALTH

WELL-BEING

BEAUTY

HOME

23. HYPERLIPIDEMIA

This is a condition in which there are high levels of fat in the blood, like cholesterol and triglycerides. Hyperlipidemia causes atherosclerosis, a disease in which plaque builds up inside the arteries, the blood vessels that carry oxygen-rich blood to the body. Plaque collects along the arterial walls and is made up of fat, cholesterol, calcium, and other substances. Over time, it hardens and makes the arterial path smaller. If not treated, blood flow can become so constricted that a heart attack, stroke, or even death may result. Atherosclerosis is a very common disease and often exists without any outward symptoms. The risk factors include an unhealthy diet, lack of exercise, and smoking. It is not surprising, then, that the main treatment is a change in lifestyle to incorporate healthy choices.

Lowering levels of fat in the blood reduces the risk of hyperlipidemia and the associated cardiovascular symptoms. To assist in this process, diffuse black cumin essential oil and inhale for one to two hours throughout the day. In hyperlipidemic rats, this oil was found to lower triglyceride levels and, in turn, lower the risk of heart disease. It also increased high density lipoprotein cholesterol levels, which reduce the risk of heart disease by removing harmful cholesterol from the blood.[42] Myrrh was also shown to lower high blood lipid levels in rats,[43] although an extract of the myrrh plant, not the essential oil, was used. The active component may be present in both the extract and the oil, giving the oil an antihyperlipidemic effect. Other essential oils used to improve cardiovascular health or help remove fats from the body are grapefruit, cinnamon leaf, ginger, peppermint, lemon, and fennel.

24. HYPERTENSION

The force exerted against arterial walls as blood flows through them determines blood pressure. The pressure is measured in the arteries when the heart contracts (systolic) and when the heart is at rest (diastolic). It is determined by how much blood the heart pumps and the resistance it encounters as it flows through the arteries. Blood pressure sustained above 140/90 mmHg (millimeters of mercury) is considered high and is called hypertension. This condition develops slowly over time, and many people have it without knowing. It can damage blood vessels and the heart. If left untreated, it can lead to heart attack and stroke. Primary hypertension doesn't have any identifiable cause, although obesity, smoking, poor diet, lack of exercise, and high salt intake are some common risk factors. Secondary hypertension has an underlying cause and could result from drugs or certain medications, alcohol abuse, thyroid problems, or kidney issues. Hypertension responds well to changes in lifestyle. Exercising more, eating a nutrient-rich diet, reducing stress, and quitting smoking and alcohol consumption should bring blood pressure down. There are many drugs available to lower blood pressure, including thiazide diuretics to reduce blood volume, beta blockers to slow down the heart rate, ACE inhibitors to block the action of some hormones that regulate blood pressure, and calcium channel blockers and renin inhibitors to widen the arteries. All these medications come with significant side effects like diarrhea, fatigue, dizziness, nausea, erectile dysfunction, and headaches.

Changes in lifestyle should be the first line of defense against high blood pressure. If additional measures are needed, try inhaling essential oils for several minutes each day before relying on any of the medications described above. Blood pressure could be lowered without having to endure any of the many side effects of conventional drugs. Hypertensive patients given a blend of lemon, lavender, and ylang-ylang essential oils to inhale twice a day for thirty days significantly lowered their systolic blood pressure and their sympathetic nerve system activity,[44] which would decrease the heart rate. Lavender and ylang-ylang can also be inhaled with bergamot essential oil to effectively reduce blood pressure from a hypertensive state.[45] Marjoram, parsley, sandalwood, yarrow, clary sage, and lemon balm are also commonly used. However, be sure to avoid hyssop, rosemary, thyme, and sage essential oils—they can negatively affect blood pressure.

25. IMMUNE SYSTEM

The immune system is the body's defense against bacteria, viruses, fungi, parasites, toxins, and allergens that could potentially invade the body and cause a lot of harm. It has a network of cells, tissues, and organs throughout the body that work around the clock and communicate when a threat is detected so it can mount a defense. Because the immune system is so busy, any help it can get is needed to prevent it from becoming overburdened. If this happens, disease can take over.

Essential oils contain different chemical compounds that can support immune function. When the body is stressed, the immune system suffers and doesn't perform optimally. Poor immune function is thought to be associated with mental health disorders like depression. When depressive patients inhaled citrus oils, neuroendocrine hormone levels returned to normal and immune function increased. This essential oil treatment was more effective than antidepressants.[46] Many oils have antifungal, antiviral, and antibacterial properties, which can attack pathogens invading the body and reduce the burden on the immune system. Laurel, sage, oregano, rosemary, and coriander were tested for their antibacterial and antifungal activity. They all showed a high degree of microbial growth inhibition, with oregano being the strongest. They also showed antioxidant activity[47] and can be used to stop free radical destruction. Free radicals are responsible for damage to cells and tissues. They are unstable molecules actively looking for an electron. Free radicals attack the nearest stable molecule and steal one of their electrons, making that molecule a free radical. This begins a chain reaction, creating free radicals that ultimately can destroy the cell. The essential oils stabilize the free radicals by giving them one of their electrons. Damage is prevented, so the immune system doesn't have to clean up the aftereffects. Some essential oils, like ylang-ylang, frankincense, marjoram, basil, cinnamon, and lemon were comparable to vitamin E and BHT, both widely used antioxidants in commercial foodstuffs.

Indian bay leaf and rose-scented geranium oil significantly decrease blood sugar levels in diabetic rats.[48, 49] This helps the liver, part of the immune system, by taking over part of its workload and allowing it to focus on its other roles. If the immune system doesn't seem to be healing wounds quickly or if multiple colds take hold over the season, it might need a little help. Dilute 2 drops of lemon oil, 2 drops of oregano oil, and 1 drop of rose-scented geranium oil in a teaspoon of grapeseed oil and massage onto the skin. Do this morning and night.

26. INDIGESTION

Indigestion is a term used to describe a feeling of fullness during a meal or an uncomfortable fullness after eating. It is often associated with pain, bloating, and burning in the stomach area. Eating too much, eating too quickly, eating certain types of food, or taking some medications can cause it. Smoking and anxiety also play a role. Sometimes, indigestion happens without any apparent reason. What causes indigestion in one person may not cause it in another. Each person needs to learn their triggers and avoid them. Even taking those measures is not enough sometimes, and medications are prescribed to find relief. Antacids, antibiotics, and antistressors can alleviate the symptoms but can also produce nausea, constipation, diarrhea, headache, abdominal pain, dizziness, weight gain, and other digestive troubles.

Ginger oil has been used as an effective and natural treatment for indigestion for many years and across many cultures. It improves bloating, relieves heartburn, and soothes pain from ulcers. Many other oils can be used to improve digestion. Clove oil reduces intestinal inflammation, relaxes muscles of the digestive tract, and reduces gas and bloating. Peppermint stimulates digestion and reduces gas pain, and the citrus oils—wild orange and lemon—relieve acid reflux. Anise, fennel, coriander, cardamom, and tarragon can also be used. Dilute 3 drops of any of these oils in a teaspoon of safflower oil and massage over the abdomen in a clockwise manner.

27. INFLAMMATION AND PAIN

Injury resulting in damaged tissue can instigate the immune system to activate the inflammatory response as part of the healing process. Foreign invaders like bacteria and viruses can likewise trigger this response to defend and rid the body of infection. White blood cells rush to the area to ingest dead or damaged cells, germs, and other foreign material. Blood flow increases and fluid leaks between cells, resulting in redness, swelling, and warmth. Pain is often associated with this process, but not always. Inflammation can be acute—sore throats, sprained ankles—or chronic—arthritis, Crohn's disease. Acute inflammation is good because it protects the body, but chronic inflammation may lead to heart problems, diabetes, cancer, and other diseases and conditions. Eating anti-inflammatory foods like cold water fish, broccoli, berries, and some whole grains and taking anti-inflammatory drugs and supplements can help.

A natural approach that can help reduce inflammation and pain locally and systemically in the body is to use essential oils. They can be applied topically to the site of inflammation or inhaled to breathe in the volatile components. *Xylopia laevigata*, a medicinal plant used in folk remedies, Mexican orange, and myrrh essential oils were tested in injury-induced rodents. They were all effective at reducing pain and inflammation.[50, 51, 52] Basil, bitter orange, black pepper, clary sage, cedarwood, clove bud, eucalyptus, foraha, fennel, ginger, helichrysum, lavender, nutmeg, pine needle, rosemary, and sage were blended together in a carrier oil and tested on their ability to reduce inflammation, ease pain, and increase mobility in rats with arthritis. Swelling was significantly reduced.[53] Pain with or without swelling can be attenuated with basil[54] and lemon essential oils.[55]

28. INSOMNIA

A good night's sleep is essential to maintain health and be produc-tive, social, and happy. Most adults require seven to eight hours a night, although it differs from person to person. Having difficulty falling asleep or staying asleep is called insomnia, and this frus-trating condition affects many people at various points throughout their lives. Insomnia can be acute and last only a night or a week, or it can be chronic and plague the sufferer for a month or longer. Stress, poor sleep habits, jet lag, night shifts, eating too much at night, medications, caffeine, nicotine, alcohol, and medical con-ditions may be responsible for keeping the mind and body from falling into a deep and restful slumber. Changing personal habits often improves insomnia. Short-term use of sleeping pills may also help, but they tend to lose their effectiveness over time. Yoga, med-itation, and acupuncture promote relaxation and can be practiced before bedtime to induce sleepiness.

Lavender is used in many products for its relaxing effects. It is no secret that new mothers are always exhausted, but trying to sleep while caring for a newborn is often difficult. A sleep study on postpartum women found that inhaling lavender essential oil at night significantly improved their quality of sleep and that this method can be used to improve maternal health.[56] Lavender oil aromatherapy increases drowsiness, promotes relaxation, and improves mood.[57] Some other oils useful at bedtime are ylang-ylang, Roman chamomile, bergamot, myrtle, sweet marjoram, and sweet thyme.[58] Sprinkle a few drops of lavender and chamomile on your pillow to inhale throughout the night.

29. IRRITABLE BOWEL SYNDROME

Irritable bowel syndrome (IBS) is a common intestinal disorder of the colon. It occurs when the muscles in the intestines contract more strongly or for longer periods of time than normal, or the contractions may be weak and slow the progression of food through the body. Abnormalities in the nervous system in the colon may also be responsible. IBS doesn't cause changes in the bowel tissue, however, and does not increase the risk of cancer like the inflammatory bowel diseases Crohn's and ulcerative colitis. It does, however, affect quality of life because the onset of symptoms can be unpredictable and come at inconvenient times, causing stress for the sufferer. Abdominal pain and cramps are often the first signs that the bowel is acting up. Diarrhea or constipation commonly follows with the expulsion of excessive gas and, sometimes, mucus in the stool. It is not uncommon to experience alternating episodes of diarrhea and constipation. IBS is chronic and cannot be cured, but symptoms often go away for periods of time, affording the person some relief. It is not known what causes irritable bowel, but each person has their own set of triggers that can cause symptoms to appear. Common triggers are particular foods, stress, hormones, and other gastrointestinal illnesses. Because the cause of IBS is unknown, changes in lifestyle are recommended to manage the condition. Learning to avoid any food triggers, decreasing stress, and taking probiotics are recommended. Doctor-prescribed medicines like antispasmodics, antidepressants, and antibiotics can treat IBS symptoms but may cause other gastrointestinal upsets, weight gain, fatigue, blurred vision, headaches, and more.

Peppermint oil shows promising use in improving the symptoms of irritable bowel syndrome. Ingestion over four weeks of sustained-release peppermint oil capsules by patients with irritable bowel syndrome found a 19.6 percent reduction of symptoms in twenty-four hours and a 40 percent reduction by the end of the study.[59] The authors state that this internal sustained release treatment is not only effective but safe. Clove oil can also be used to reduce intestinal inflammation, relax muscles of the digestive tract, and reduce gas and bloating. Other oils to combine with peppermint are ginger, geranium, fennel, marjoram, and rose.

30. ITCHY SKIN

Itchy skin can be very uncomfortable and make you want to scratch. Itches can be localized to a specific area or generalized and occur all over the body. One of the most common causes is simply dry skin, and this is easily improved by adding moisture with creams, lotions, and oils. Other causes cannot be resolved so easily. These include itch from allergic reactions, medications, diseases, emotional issues, and skin conditions like eczema. Sometimes itchy skin is accompanied by bumps, rashes, blisters, or red and inflamed skin. Scratching the itch provides temporary relief but can injure the skin, causing it to look red, feel raw, and, in some cases, become inflamed and bleed. This can lead to infection. Anti-itch creams and lotions can temporarily dull the itch, and cold compresses can quiet the nerve fibers, since cold and itching travel along the same nerves.

Over-the-counter products containing menthol and camphor are often used to temporarily relieve itch. Rather than using these commercial products that contain a number of other often undesirable chemicals, find comfort through diffusing the pure essential oils of white camphor and peppermint and inhaling their aroma for periods throughout the day. Oils can also be applied topically, directly to the skin, to soothe itch. A study using a 5 percent solution of mint, lavender, and tea tree oils was massaged on the arms of hemodialysis patients suffering from itchy skin. Itchiness significantly decreased.[60] Some others to use for their anti-inflammatory, antiseptic, or soothing qualities—all of which help calm itch—are Roman chamomile, lavender, patchouli, tea tree, myrrh, palmarosa, and sandalwood.

31. JET LAG

The whole world has become much more accessible to travelers. Visiting places all over the globe is a reality in which many choose to partake. With travel across time zones, the body is forced to alter its internal clock that tells us when to sleep and when to be awake.

HEALTH

WELL-BEING

BEAUTY

HOME

HEALTH

WELL-BEING

BEAUTY

HOME

This doesn't happen spontaneously, and the body needs a period of time to adjust. What results is jet lag. Sleep is often disturbed, and many have trouble falling asleep or wake too early. During the day, symptoms of fatigue, moodiness, gastrointestinal issues, and poor concentration are commonly felt. Although jet lag is temporary and recovery is complete after a few days, travelers sometimes turn to sleeping pills. While these do increase the duration of sleep, they don't generally lessen fatigue during the day. Melatonin, caffeine drinks, and light therapy are other popular alternatives to induce sleep or increase alertness.

Essential oils can both stimulate and relax the mind and body. When it is time to sleep, inhale lavender oil or sprinkle a few drops on your pillow before resting. This oil increases drowsiness, elevates mood, and encourages relaxation.[61] Some other oils useful at bedtime are ylang-ylang, Roman chamomile, bergamot, myrtle, marjoram, and sweet thyme.[62] During the day, replace the lavender oil with rosemary oil to maintain a relaxed mood but increase alertness.[63] If renting a car to do some sightseeing, add rosemary oil to a cotton ball and place between two slats in one of the car's air vents. This will disperse the scent throughout the car. Pine, eucalyptus, peppermint, grapefruit, and basil oils can be used in place of, or in addition to, rosemary essential oil.

32. LARYNGITIS

The larynx, also known as the voice box, houses the vocal cords, which vibrate when air is passed through them, and produces sound. Laryngitis is when the vocal cords become inflamed, resulting in hoarseness or loss of voice. This condition can be acute, coming on suddenly from a viral infection or overuse, and lasts no more than a few weeks. Chronic laryngitis can also be caused by an infection, but exposure to inhaled irritants, chronic sinusitis, acid reflux, inhaled steroid medications, and excessive coughing are other sources. This type of laryngitis can last three weeks or longer, depending on how long the larynx is exposed to the irritating conditions or chemicals. Those with symptoms lasting longer than two weeks should consult a doctor, but acute cases can be treated at home with vocal rest.

Essential oils can alleviate the symptoms of a sore throat and allow a speedy recovery. Using oils that have anti-inflammatory and antimicrobial properties will soothe the vocal tissues, reduce swelling, and help eliminate any infection responsible for this condition. Add 2 to 3 drops of Roman chamomile and lavender oils into a bowl containing hot water. Drape a towel over your head and inhale the steam for five minutes. Try adding a few drops of geranium, niaouli, sage, pine, lemon, or ginger oils to warm water and dip a washcloth into it. Squeeze out the excess water and lay the cloth across your larynx. These oils can be diffused, too, but make sure to do it in a steamy room, like the bathroom with the shower on. The moisture helps break up the mucus in the throat.

33. LICE

Every year, it seems children are sent home from school with a note warning parents that there is an outbreak of head lice in the school. These tiny insects that infest children's (and adults') scalps

HEALTH

WELL-BEING

BEAUTY

HOME

are a source of panic and embarrassment, although having lice is not a sign of poor personal hygiene. They can fall off the head and land on the carpet, bedding, towels, and stuffed animals where they lay their eggs and continue to grow for another day or two. Lice feed on the blood of the scalp and are readily transferred from one person to another through direct contact. A person may be infected for several weeks before itching begins. The itching is an allergic reaction to the louse saliva. The lice and nits (eggs) are difficult to see, but a close look around the ears and neckline may provide the best chance of glimpsing them. Over-the-counter and prescription medicated shampoos are used to kill the adult lice. The eggs are hard to get rid of, though, because they adhere to the hair shaft with a sticky substance that is difficult to wash out. A second treatment of medicated shampoo is recommended when the nits hatch.

A study was undertaken on the efficacy of using a tea tree oil and lavender oil treatment on killing live lice. This was compared to a product that suffocates the lice and a third treatment containing commonly used pesticidal compounds. The tea tree oil and lavender oil treatment eliminated 97.6 percent of the lice, the same as the suffocation treatment, and was significantly higher than the pesticidal treatment.[64] This essential oil combination was also found to be 44.4 percent effective at eliminating the eggs of the lice as well[65] and is recommended as a first line of treatment for lice infestations.

34. LISTERIOSIS

Listeriosis is a serious infection caused by eating food contaminated with the bacteria *Listeria monocytogenes*. These bacteria are contracted by humans most commonly through deli meats, hot dogs, unpasteurized milk, and soft cheeses. Most people who come into contact with these bacteria are not seriously affected and may experience muscle aches, headaches, nausea, and diarrhea. Pregnant mothers need to be very vigilant during pregnancy because *Listeria* can be life threatening to the fetus or newborn baby. People with weakened immune systems are also at higher risk of developing serious or life-threatening complications. This illness usually runs its course without intervention, but in high-risk patients, antibiotics are commonly prescribed.

A 2 percent solution of clove oil and lemongrass oil (96 drops of essential oils to 1 cup of water) can be sprayed on paper towels and wrapped around soft cheeses, hot dogs, and deli meats to prevent the growth of *Listeria* bacteria. Research was performed on the ability of these oils to inhibit the growth of *Listeria monocytogenes* in bovine ground meat. At concentrations of 1.56 percent, these oils significantly reduced bacterial populations after one day.[66] Combining the use of these oils with other measures, such as refrigeration of meats, cheeses, and milk, can help control the growth of these bacteria and increase food shelf life.

HEALTH

WELL-BEING

BEAUTY

HOME

35. LIVER DAMAGE FROM TOXINS

The liver is the largest internal organ in the body. It filters toxins out of the bloodstream to prevent them from damaging tissues. When the liver tissue itself becomes damaged, it has the ability to regenerate and make new, healthy tissue. However, prolonged or acute toxin exposure can overwhelm the liver so that it doesn't have the capability to heal itself. Normal functioning is obstructed, and the toxins can attack other tissues, causing systemic implications. Symptoms include upper right abdominal pain, nausea, vomiting, fatigue, loss of appetite, and jaundice. It's imperative to stop exposure to toxins before the damage becomes irreversible.

Toxic chemicals can be found all around us. A few places they are lurking are in cleaning products, flame retardants, air fresheners, nonstick cookware, and bug sprays. The liver has a big job in trying to neutralize all these before they cause damage to the body. Marjoram essential oil provides protection against prallethrin, a chemical compound found in insecticides. A study in male rats fed prallethrin found that when marjoram essential oil was co-administered with the insecticide, the toxic effect was lowered. Liver injury and oxidative damage was minimized.[67] Helichrysum can be used to boost liver function too, as can Roman chamomile, cypress, and carrot seed oils. Other oils can help detoxify the body to aid in the liver's recovery. These include peppermint, lemon, tea tree, rosemary, grapefruit, and juniper berry.

36. MENSTRUAL PAIN

Women of childbearing years often experience pain and cramping just before or during the first few days of menstruation. Pain can be mild to severe and is described as a dull, throbbing ache in the lower abdomen, hips, back, and thighs. It usually lasts twelve to seventy-two hours and, for some, can prevent normal activities for several days. It happens when the muscles of the woman's uterus contract too strongly and put pressure on nearby blood vessels. Oxygen to muscle tissue of the uterus is temporarily cut off, and pain results. Over-the-counter pain relievers and hormone birth control are used to relieve pain. Primary menstrual cramps usually occur each menstrual cycle and can be associated with other symptoms like nausea, vomiting, diarrhea, and fatigue. They are differentiated from secondary menstrual pain, which has an underlying cause like a reproductive disorder or infection. The main objective in managing this condition is to reduce pain and treat the symptoms.

A study testing the pain-mitigating effects of a cream composed of 3 percent lavender, clary sage, and marjoram essential oils found that the duration of menstrual pain was significantly reduced.[68] A similar study found that a combination of lavender, clary sage, and rose essential oils decreases the severity of menstrual pain.[69] Other oils to reduce pain are geranium, Roman chamomile, and eucalyptus. Some do double duty. Ylang-ylang acts as a sedative and antispasmodic, peppermint and ginger oils can reduce pain and nausea, and black pepper and cypress minimize pain and bloating.

To relieve the duration and intensity of pain and other symptoms during menstruation, massage 1 teaspoon of almond oil containing 2 drops of lavender and 1 drop of peppermint essential oils onto the abdominal area. Begin one day before the onset of menstruation and continue for several days after. Select oils that will benefit specific symptoms.

37. NAUSEA

Nausea can be caused by a number of situations, conditions, or diseases. Motion sickness from up-and-down, side-to-side, or circular and jerky movements can cause severe dizziness, cold sweats, nausea, and vomiting. This illness can happen during any type of motion, including travel by air, boat, car, or train. It happens when the signals received from the eyes, the body, and the inner ear send conflicting messages to the brain. Morning sickness induces nausea and vomiting in pregnancy and is most likely a result of hormonal changes in the body. Chemotherapy evokes the same in patients, depending on which drugs are received, dosages, and whether chemotherapy is used in conjunction with other therapies such as radiation. Drugs, supplements, and even stress and anxiety can increase the risk of nausea and, once started, is difficult to control. Antinausea medications are often prescribed in pill or patch form, but there are a wide variety of side effects that can lead to drowsiness, dry mouth, headache, muscle pain, diarrhea, constipation, blurred vision, and disorientation.

Peppermint has traditionally been used to reduce nausea from motion sickness. Carry a cotton ball with a few drops of peppermint essential oil on it and inhale when feeling nauseated. Results should be immediate. Peppermint oil has also been shown to reduce nausea postoperatively[70] and can lower or even eliminate the use of antinausea medication. Ginger, spearmint, and sweet orange essential oils can dispel morning sickness, while cardamom can be used to attenuate nausea from chemotherapy. An easy way to get the benefits of these oils when you're feeling low is to diffuse them and allow the room to fill with the aroma. All you need to do is breathe in.

38. NERVE PAIN

Nerve pain can result from diseased or damaged nerves of the peripheral nervous system. Communication between the brain and the affected parts of the body is interrupted and can result in numbness or tingling in the hands and feet, muscle weakness or lack of coordination, sensitivity to touch, and pain. Damage to the nerves can be a result of toxic exposure, injury, medications, nutritional deficiencies, inherited conditions, or diseases, such as diabetes. Pain-relieving medications, surgery, physical therapy, transcutaneous electrical nerve stimulation, and acupuncture are all used to try to reduce nerve pain.

Nerves have the capability to heal themselves if the damage is not too severe. This is a slow process that can take up to nine months or longer. It is essential to find the source of the nerve pain before healing can begin. In the meantime, pain management is the priority. Surgery should always be a last option, and taking drugs, while effective in many, has a long list of undesirable side effects. Using essential oils to curb pain can be effective and safe for the recovering body. The topical treatment of peppermint oil applied to the skin of a woman suffering from nerve pain was immediately effective in reducing nerve pain. The effect lasted four to six hours after application.[71] Another study on neuropathic pain found that lavender, geranium, bergamot, tea tree, and eucalyptus oils blended with six homeopathic substances reduced pain in 93.3 percent of subjects within thirty minutes. This result was significantly higher than the placebo group that saw an improvement in only 35 percent of subjects.[72] Roman chamomile, West Indian bay, sweet marjoram, ginger, and black pepper are other essential oils used to soothe nerve pain. Add a few drops to a teaspoon of rice bran oil and then pour into a warm bath or massage onto the skin for immediate and lasting relief.

39. ORAL THRUSH

When the yeast *C. albicans* overgrows in the lining of the mouth, white lesions develop on the tongue and inner cheeks and may cause redness and soreness. This is called thrush. While *Candida* are normally present in the body, their numbers are kept in check by the immune system. Sometimes, when the immune system is weakened by disease or drugs, *Candida* grows out of control and causes an infection. It is most common in babies and the elderly but is also seen in adults with compromised immune systems. This condition is not generally serious, but if left unchecked, the yeast can spread to other areas of the body like the lungs, heart, liver, and digestive tract. Most cases are controlled with antifungal medications.

Lavender essential oil inhibits the growth of both the yeast and hyphal forms of *C. albicans*[73] and can be used to reduce the spread of infection. Clove oil and thyme oil also demonstrate antifungal activity against *Candida*.[74] The active ingredients are eugenol, which is also found in cinnamon, nutmeg, basil, vanilla, oregano, dill, and lemon balm essential oils, and thymus, also found in bergamot. Make an oral solution containing a teaspoon of virgin coconut oil—which also has anti-*Candida* activity—with 3 drops of any of the antifungal oils and swish around the mouth for several minutes. Spit in the garbage when finished.

40. PANCREATIC CANCER

Pancreatic cancer begins in the tissues of the pancreas, the organ that lies horizontally behind the lower part of the stomach. The pancreas secretes enzymes to aid in digestion and hormones to regulate the metabolism of sugars. Cancer develops when cells mutate and grow rapidly and continuously. They live long after normal pancreatic cells have died and eventually form into tumors. This disease often goes undetected and spreads rapidly. Symptoms begin to appear later in its progression and may include loss of appetite, weight loss, blood clots, depression, upper abdominal pain, and jaundice. Treatment options are surgery, chemotherapy, and radiation.

Frankincense essential oil was tested against human pancreatic cancer cell lines and showed potential as an alternative therapeutic candidate for treating patients with this aggressive type of cancer. The oil stopped the cancer cell's growth and activated the pathway leading to cell death.[75] Patients can add this to their treatment plan

HEALTH

WELL-BEING

BEAUTY

HOME

by diffusing the oil into the air and breathing deeply. For a topical application, 3 drops of the oil can be added to a teaspoon of argan oil and poured into a warm bath or massaged over the abdomen.

41. PERINEAL RELIEF (AFTER CHILDBIRTH)

Childbirth through vaginal delivery stretches the vagina and can lead to postpartum pain in the perineum (the tissue between the vagina and the anus). Even women who have cesarean sections following long labors may experience such pain. About half of women tear the perineal tissue as the baby pushes through and require stitches. This extends healing time, and the area will be tender and sore. The tissue should heal within ten days, but the pain may persist for weeks longer. Keeping the area clean and using fresh maxi pads every four to six hours will help. Applying cold packs, taking warm baths, and using donut-shaped cushions will be beneficial as well.

Following childbirth, women who added lavender essential oil to their baths reported less discomfort between the third and fifth days compared to women using synthetic lavender oil or a placebo oil.[76] Lavender oil can be added to warm water in a squirt bottle and used to clean the area after urinating to help speed recovery and improve comfort. In addition, add a few drops of Roman chamomile and tea tree essential oils to a cool sitz bath along with some bath salts (dissolve the bath salts in warm water first). This will promote wound healing and reduce inflammation and pain. Do this two to three times a day. In between baths, apply to the perineum a cold maxi pad that was dipped in water containing basil and helichrysum essential oils before freezing. These oils will help reduce pain, protect against infection, and heal the perineal tissue.

42. PERIoDONTITIS

It is extremely important to have a good oral hygiene routine to prevent periodontitis. This is a serious gum disease in which the gums pull away from the teeth and form pockets where bacteria can breed and cause inflammation. The pockets become deeper, allowing more bacteria to accumulate. Inflammation worsens, and infection sets in. Eventually the gums, tissue, and bones that support the teeth are destroyed, and the teeth may fall out or need to be removed. Be on the lookout for gums that are red, swollen, and tender to the touch. New spaces may develop between the teeth, and they could begin to feel loose. If this happens or if the gums recede or pus is found between the teeth and gums, it is time to take action and see a dentist to stop the progression of this disease.

Black sage essential oil was administered to rats with periodontitis three times a day for eleven days. Compared to the placebo oil, black sage inhibited bone loss and the growth of *P. gingivalis*, an oral bacteria that contributes to periodontitis.[77] A few drops of black sage essential oil can be combined with a teaspoon of virgin coconut oil—also great for destroying bacteria in the mouth—and swished around the mouth for twenty minutes before spitting out in the garbage. Do this once a day for improved oral health. Other antibacterial oils to use are clove, peppermint, oregano, orange, cinnamon leaf, and lavender. These oils can be diluted 1:4 in virgin coconut oil and rubbed over the gums.

43. PNEUMONIA

Pneumonia is an infection of the lungs that causes inflammation of the air sacs, which may fill with pus or fluid. Different bacteria, viruses, and fungi can cause pneumonia when a person breathes in air containing the pathogens. In hospital settings, the bacteria *Klebsiella pneumoniae* is often a cause of pneumonia in patients whose immune systems are already compromised due to other illnesses. Here, it is most commonly spread by patient-to-patient contact, ventilation machines, or catheters. If acquired, the patient may experience chest pain, shortness of breath, cough with phlegm, nausea, fever, and fatigue. This type of pneumonia can be very serious, not only because the patients have a harder time fighting the bacterial infection on their own but because this type of bacteria tends to be resistant to antibiotics.

Eugenol is a compound found in many essential oils including clove, bay leaf, geranium, oregano, nutmeg, cinnamon, basil, dill, and lemon balm. This compound was tested against the pneumonia-causing *Klebsiella pneumoniae* bacteria and was found to inhibit its growth, whereas the antibiotics ampicillin, erythromycin, and sulfamethizole were unable to do so.[78] Add a few drops of clove, nutmeg, and lemon balm oils to warm water in a bowl. Lean over the bowl and cover the head with a towel. Breathe deeply. Inhaling these volatile oils should allow the eugenol to enter the lungs and work on the bacteria at the site of infection.

44. POISON IVY

A lucky 15 percent of the population is not allergic to poison ivy. That means 85 percent need to be extra cautious when outdoors in areas known to have the plant. Brushing up against the leaves, stems, or roots of the plant can transfer an oily resin called urushiol to the skin. Even if direct contact with the plant wasn't made, touching pets, gardening tools, clothing, or other items that contacted the plant can transfer the urushiol. The resin quickly penetrates the skin, and symptoms develop within twelve to seventy-two hours. Redness, itching, swelling, and blisters that may weep and crust over are commonly found on the skin and last anywhere from one to three weeks. The rash is not contagious, but urushiol can be transferred from person to person. Washing the affected skin with mild soap and warm water to remove the resin will lessen the severity of the infection or even prevent it if the resin is washed away before it has a chance to penetrate the skin. Poison ivy is self-limiting and often goes away on its own, but if it is severe or an infection starts, corticosteroids and antibiotics are prescribed by a doctor.

Manuka, mullein, sage, rose, sandalwood, and yarrow are just a few helpful essential oils that can reduce the inflammation and itch caused by the poison ivy allergic rash. Reducing swelling will lessen the pressure on the nerves and stop the itch sensation.

Mexican orange and myrrh essential oils were tested and found to be effective at reducing pain and inflammation.[79, 80] A blend of basil, bitter orange, black pepper, clary sage, cedarwood, clove bud, eucalyptus, foraha, fennel, ginger, helichrysum, lavender, nutmeg, pine needle, rosemary, and sage essential oils also reduced inflammation and eased pain in laboratory tests on rats.[81] Tea tree, peppermint, lavender, oregano, patchouli, and cypress oils applied to the skin can be used to prevent bacteria from infecting the injured skin. Add a few drops of peppermint oil to a teaspoon of aloe vera gel for this purpose to ease itching and inflammation and protect against infection. To promote growth and regeneration of new cells during the skin's healing phase, take a warm bath using manuka, tea tree, and lavender essential oils.

45. RINGWORM

Worms do not actually cause this condition. Ringworm is a fungal infection of the outer layers of skin that is characterized by a red rash that forms a circle—or ring—on the surface of the skin with a clearer patch of skin in the middle. The fungus can affect any area of the body with one or many rings. It is contagious and is spread from one infected person or animal to another. Even touching bedding, towels, or surfaces that were in contact with the fungus can cause it to adhere to the skin and begin to multiply. Children are most susceptible. Initially, the rash is red, itchy, and flat. If it progresses, the skin can become inflamed with pus-filled blisters. Over-the-counter fungal creams can be used to get rid of the infection, but in severe cases, prescription antifungal medications may be needed.

A popular home remedy to treat the fungus causing ringworm is tea tree oil. This essential oil contains antifungal compounds that inhibit the growth of the fungi.[82] Make a strong dilution of one fourth tea tree oil to three fourths virgin coconut oil. Clean and dry the ringworm-infected area and apply the oil mixture directly to the skin with a cotton ball. Be sure to throw the cotton ball away after use to prevent reuse and reinfection. Do this three times a day for several weeks or until the infection has cleared. At night, put a thicker layer of the mixture over the skin, cover with a wrap, and secure. Mixing tea tree oil with coconut oil will provide different methods to attack the fungi because coconut oil is also an effective ringworm antifungal.

46. SCABIES

For over 2500 years, scabies infestations have been plaguing humans of every race and age. It is estimated that over 300 million cases of scabies are contracted worldwide each year from the highly contagious itch mite, *Sarcoptes scabiei*. This mite is spread by direct person-to-person contact and, once on the skin, burrows into it and produces an allergic reaction, manifesting as extremely itchy, small red bumps and blisters. The itch is relentless and tends to be worse at night, affecting sleep. Excessive scratching sometimes leads to secondary infections. These symptoms may not be evident for a few months, but the mites can still be spread during this time. After diagnosis, a cream containing a mite killer, like permethrin, or an oral medication, like ivermectin, is prescribed. The cream is applied from the neck down and left on overnight before being washed off. A second treatment is needed in seven days. Alternative treatments are available, but they are not all approved by the FDA and come with serious side effects. Antihistamines can also be taken to reduce inflammation and itch.

Tea tree oil has shown to be effective in eliminating scabies mites and is superior to the commonly used scabicidal treatments of permethrin and ivermectin.[83] Tea tree oil has antibacterial properties that can help prevent secondary infections from establishing themselves in the injured skin and is thought to reduce inflammation and itching. Use this as a topical treatment for scabies by diluting 5 drops of essential oil in virgin coconut oil and apply to the rash. Other antibacterial and anti-inflammatory oils that can help reduce swelling and prevent secondary infections include white camphor, Roman chamomile, eucalyptus, rose, sage, sandalwood, and yarrow.

47. SEIZURES

Abnormal electrical activity in the brain can cause seizures. Anything that affects the body can also affect the brain, so seizures can be initiated by alcohol, drugs, medications, allergic reactions, head injuries, fever, and stroke. Some cause uncontrollable shaking or convulsions, while others are less obvious and may look like the person is unfocused and staring into space. They can affect one side of the brain (and body) or both sides and usually last from thirty seconds to several minutes. While most seizures do not have lasting harmful effects, it's important to see a doctor to determine if there is an underlying cause. Treatment for seizures vary but include medications, nerve stimulation, surgery, and changes in diet.

Anise essential oil has been traditionally used to treat some neurological disorders. A study in epileptic rats found that anise oil has antiseizure and neuroprotective effects, possibly by inhibiting the transmission of signals along nerves. This oil also suppressed the formation of dark neurons in different parts of the brain, meaning the oil protected the brain's neurons from damage and death during the seizures.[84] If prone to seizures, use anise regularly. Pregnant women and those with estrogen-dependent cancers should avoid it.

48. SMOKING WITHDRAWAL

Cigarettes and other tobacco products contain the addictive drug nicotine. Up to 90 percent of people who smoke regularly become addicted to nicotine, making it very difficult to stop. Once in the body, nicotine gets into the bloodstream and travels to the brain within fifteen seconds. Here, chemicals are released that produce a happy, relaxed feeling. Adrenaline is also released and increases heart rate and blood pressure. With continued use, nicotine damages the lungs, arteries, and heart. It increases the risk of heart attack, stroke, lung disease, osteoporosis, and cancer. It weakens the immune system. It negatively affects eyesight and causes erectile dysfunction. The list goes on, and it is vitally important to stop using nicotine to restore health. Withdrawal usually lasts from a few days to a few weeks and can make you feel unwell.

Besides willpower, currently available treatments include nicotine replacement therapy, medications to reduce withdrawal symptoms, counseling, hypnosis, and acupuncture. Essential oils also have a role to play in eliminating cravings and helping to reduce withdrawal symptoms. Vapor inhalation of black pepper essential oil reduced cravings for cigarettes compared to inhalation of menthol or plain air. The intensity of sensation from inhaling black pepper oil was significantly higher, which is important in reducing smoking withdrawal symptoms.[85] Others use clary sage, patchouli, and spikenard. Adding Roman chamomile, ylang-ylang, or bergamot oils to the others can help reduce anxiety during this time and mimic the happy, relaxed feeling smoking can bring. When cravings strike, inhale a blend of black pepper and bitter orange. A few drops of each of these oils can be placed on a cotton ball and kept close by.

49. STAPHYL°COCCUS INFECTION

There are over thirty types of bacterial *Staphylococcus* (staph) infections, but most are caused by *Staphylococcus aureus* (*S. aureus*). These bacteria are responsible for skin infections, pneumonia, food poisoning, blood poisoning, and toxic shock syndrome. Staph skin infections are most common and are usually minor. They look like pimples, blisters, or boils. More severe infections, however, can show red, swollen rashes with pus or drainage. Many people carry these bacteria on their skin or in their noses without any symptoms. The bacteria get into the skin through cuts or scrapes, so it is important to keep wounds clean and to wash hands regularly. If the bacteria invade the body and get into the bloodstream, infections can turn up in numerous organs and become life threatening. Treatment for minor staph infections is usually a course of antibiotics or drainage of infected areas. Severe infections require hospitalization. Many varieties of staph have become resistant to antibiotics. New treatments are needed to continue to fight these ubiquitous bacteria.

The bactericidal activity of some essential oils is potent enough to inhibit the growth of staph infections, including those demonstrating antibiotic resistance. Tea tree essential oil is one of these and has been shown to inhibit the growth of *S. aureus*.[86] It was found to be as effective as standard treatment regimens and more effective than commercial topical antiseptics at eliminating staph skin infections.[87] Grapefruit seed oil and geranium oil used in combination are also highly effective at clearing antibiotic-resistant staph infections.[88] Lavender, peppermint, thyme,[89] Turkish oregano, Damask rose, Greek juniper, and chrysanthemum oils[90] can also be used with success. For skin infections, apply a topical solution of 2 drops of tea tree oil and 1 drop of geranium oil in 1 teaspoon of virgin coconut oil. All three oils work against *S. aureus*.

50. SuN FUNGUS (TINEA VERSICOLoR)

This condition is caused by the fungus *Malassezia* that resides on the skin. When it grows out of control and causes an infection, it affects the normal pigmentation of the skin, resulting in patches that are lighter or darker than normal. It can cause some mild itching and scaling and becomes more noticeable with sun exposure. It is not known precisely why such infections begin, but hot and humid weather, oily skin, hormonal changes, or a compromised immune system are contributing factors. This condition is not contagious and is found mostly in teenagers and young adults. Oral or topical over-the-counter antifungal medications can be used to return the skin to normal, but severe infections will likely require different medications prescribed by doctors. Pigmentation should return to normal after several weeks or months, but be aware that this infection may return and medications will be needed again.

The antifungal activity of tea tree essential oil was tested against *Malassezia* strains and found to be effective in reducing fungal numbers.[91] Tea tree oil is safe to use on the skin, so making a more concentrated solution of this oil in a carrier oil is acceptable and may provide enhanced activity against sun fungus. Add 10 drops of tea tree oil to a teaspoon of jojoba oil and massage into the affected areas of the skin. Do this twice a day until you feel the infection has cleared. Remember, even after fungal growth has stopped, the skin pigmentation will take some time to return to normal.

51. VAGINAL YEAST INFECTION

Vaginal yeast infections are caused most often by the *Candida albicans* fungus. It is very common, affecting up to 75 percent of women at some point in their lives. This fungus normally lives in the vagina in small numbers, but sometimes when conditions change to affect the balance of microorganisms, *Candida* grows in numbers, creating an infection. Imbalances can be created from antibiotics, hormonal changes, pregnancy, diabetes, a weakened immune system, too much sugary food in the diet, and stress. Once established, this infection can cause abnormal vaginal discharge, inflammation of vaginal tissue, painful urination, itching, and burning. Over-the-counter antifungal medications can clear the infection within two weeks. These infections have a high recurrence rate, and medications will need to be taken each time.

The essential oil of apple mint can be used to help treat vaginal yeast infections. This oil demonstrated potent antifungal activity against *Candida albicans* in laboratory experiments and was able to speed up the process of clearing the infection in mice with chronic vaginal candidiasis.[92] Lavender oil inhibits *Candida albicans* growth and was able to kill 100 percent of one strain in fifteen minutes.[93] Other oils effective in inhibiting *Candida* fungal growth include narrow-leaved paperbark,[94] clove, geranium, oregano, nutmeg, dill, lemon balm, bay leaf, basil, tea tree, and cinnamon leaf. These oils remove the source of infection and reduce pain, redness, and inflammation. Fill a sitz bath with cool water and add about twenty drops of apple mint and tea tree oils. Sit and relax in the bath for twenty minutes, allowing the solution to wash in and around the vagina. Do this twice a day for a week. In between baths, dilute 3 drops of any of these oils in a teaspoon of virgin coconut oil and apply to the inflamed tissue outside the vagina.

52. WEIGHT LOSS

When the body accumulates too much body fat, it increases the risk of health problems like diabetes, heart disease, and certain cancers. Losing weight can improve or prevent any weight-induced conditions. Losing weight means losing fat, which accumulates on the body when more calories are eaten than burned. The body stores these excess calories as fat. Exercising and eating a healthy diet with appropriate calorie intake will help burn the stored fat and reduce body weight.

Inhaling citronella oil decreased body weight in male rats fed a high-fat diet over five weeks compared to the control group of rats who did not inhale the oil. It was found that the rats inhaling citronella oil had decreased appetite and consumed fewer calories.[95] Peppermint, grapefruit, and fennel oils can improve weight loss efforts by suppressing food cravings. Grapefruit oil also boosts energy for sustained calorie-burning exercise. Ginger oil is thermogenic, meaning it burns calories by converting them into heat. Eating foods that encourage the body to produce heat can increase metabolism by as much as 5 percent and fat-burning potential by as much as 16 percent.[96] Lemongrass is also thought to be a thermogenic oil. Dilute these oils in apricot kernel oil and dab on the bottom of the feet. The wrists are another good place and can be inhaled periodically.

53. WOUND ODOR

Offensive odors can arise from pressure ulcers, diabetic foot ulcers, leg ulcers, or other skin lesions on the body. These odors can be foul to anyone within close proximity to the patient, but the effects on the patients themselves can be devastating. They may withdraw socially, reject intimacy, and feel nauseated or lose their appetite. These wounds can become host to many different microbes, which thrive on necrotic tissue and emit compounds that generate the repellant smell. Doctors can prescribe systemic or topical antibiot-ics to treat the infection, but routine use is discouraged because of bacterial resistance problems and patient sensitivities.

Malodorous wounds are notoriously difficult to treat, and cur-rent medications cannot reduce the smell to acceptable levels. Cancer patients receiving standard antibiotics for necrotic ulcers also had an antibacterial essential oil mix rinsed over the ulcers twice a day. Eucalyptus oil was the primary essential oil in the mix. One hundred percent of patients achieved complete elimination of the smell by the third or fourth day of treatment. The oils also reduced inflammation of the wounds, and some patients saw their ulcers begin to heal. Quality of life for these patients significantly improved.[97]

HEALTH

WELL-BEING

BEAUTY

HOME

CHAPTER 2

....

RESTORING MENTAL AND EMOTIONAL WELL-BEING

....

54. ANGER

Anger is a normal human emotion that can and should be dealt with but, in some, gets out of control and becomes disruptive or dangerous. Anger can range from mild irritation to outright fury. As this emotion becomes more intense, the body responds by increasing heart rate, blood pressure, adrenaline, and noradrenaline. This can be perilous for those with hypertension or heart conditions. Dealing with anger requires expressing it in an assertive, nonthreatening way, suppressing it and refocusing that energy into positive activities or thoughts, or calming down both outward reactions and internal responses like heart rate, blood pressure, and feelings of depression.

Aromatherapy uses essential oils to enhance physical and emotional well-being. Inhaling these aromatic oils sends messages from the smell receptors in the nose to the part of the brain responsible for emotions and behavior. This part is also connected to other parts of the brain that control breathing, blood pressure, stress, memory, and hormones.[98] Massaging essential oils into the skin allows the unique active components of the oil to penetrate the skin or other tissues within twenty minutes[99] and even cross the blood-brain barrier. Some oils have a very calming effect on the brain and body and can be used in times of anger, frustration, and irritation to reduce the intensity of these feelings. Frankincense, rose, lemon, sweet orange, grapefruit, sweet marjoram, and vetiver are wonderfully calming oils. Make a spritz using 1/2 cup distilled water, 1 tablespoon witch hazel, 2 drops frankincense, 2 drops sweet orange, and 2 drops vetiver essential oils. Shake well before use. When feelings of anger begin to overwhelm, spritz one or two times and inhale.

55. ANXIETY

Everyone feels anxiety at certain times in their life. Before going on a job interview, stepping out on a first date, or moving to a new city, you may experience fear, worry, nervousness, panic, or uneasiness. These feelings usually subside after the event has passed. For some, these feelings don't resolve and are persistent and overwhelming. This is another level of anxiety and is classified as an anxiety disorder. There are different types, but they can all interfere with normal life and be so intense and disabling that the afflicted withdraw from society. Anxiety is caused by changes in the functioning of the part of the brain that regulates emotions. On a physiological level, the person may have shortness of breath, heart palpitations, nausea, muscle tension, and insomnia. Drugs can be used to reduce symptoms, counseling to address emotional issues, diet changes to improve overall body function, and relaxation techniques to self-soothe.

Some people with anxiety do require the help of doctors and counselors to assist them in dealing with psychological issues and physical symptoms. It does not matter if anxiety stems from normal fear and worry or from a diagnosed anxiety disorder; essential oils have the ability to affect the limbic system of the brain that controls emotions and can be used to reduce these negative feelings. A study in mice found that bitter orange essential oil significantly reduced anxiety, likely by having an effect on the 5-HT_{1A} receptor in the brain that controls mood.[100] Another study in female hemodialysis patients found that inhaling hiba and lavender essential oils were effective in reducing anxiety during their treatments.[101] Rosemary oil and Roman chamomile oil have also been studied and found to reduce anxiety.[102, 103] Other oils to use are bergamot, frankincense, sweet marjoram, neroli, patchouli, angelica seed, and ylang-ylang. For the best release of anxiety, draw a warm bath and add a few drops each of clary sage, rose, and Roman chamomile. Relax in the bath for twenty minutes.

56. CONCENTRATION

Concentration is the ability to keep the mind focused on an activity for a desired period of time. It seems that some people are able to concentrate on a task for several hours, yet for others, their attention begins to wane after only a few minutes. Some medical conditions interfere with the ability to concentrate, as do psychological and cognitive problems. Poor concentration may be a symptom of something else, so seeing a trained professional is important if an underlying reason for an inability to concentrate is suspected. For many, however, concentration can seem to slip as they get older and find themselves getting bored and distracted or slipping away into daydreams. A growing body of science points to two regions in the frontal lobes of the brain that gradually shift into a seesaw imbalance with age and, with it, a decreased ability to concentrate on the task at hand. This shift begins in middle age and becomes more pronounced in older adults.[104]

There are many essential oils that have antioxidative capabilities. Some of the most powerful ones are clove, myrrh, citronella, coriander, fennel, and clary sage. They stop free radicals in the brain from oxidizing other molecules by donating one of their extra electrons to the free radical to stabilize it, preventing premature aging, damage, and impairment of brain cell function. Regularly using these essential oils can prevent loss of concentration due to free radical damage. For an immediate boost to improve focus, place 2 drops of peppermint and 2 drops of grapefruit essential oils in a diffuser and inhale. Rosemary and sweet orange or eucalyptus, lemon, and patchouli oils can be used as well.

57. DEPRESSION

Depression is a mood disorder that causes a deep sadness and a loss of interest in activities. It affects how a person feels, thinks, and behaves and can cause not just emotional problems but can also manifest as physical problems. Clinical depression may occur once in a person's lifetime or reoccur multiple times. This feeling of sadness and loss can cause insomnia, loss of appetite, poor concentration, fatigue, suicidal thoughts, and physical symptoms like backaches and headaches. Changes in the body's hormone levels may cause or trigger depression. Modifications to the way brain chemicals work and the effect that has on maintaining stable moods is thought to play a major role. Psychological counseling and antidepressant medications are often prescribed. Antidepressants can cause a wide range of side effects, including nausea, insomnia, blurred vision, weight gain, fatigue, and sexual dysfunction.

When neuroendocrine hormone levels are off balance, mood is affected and depression may result. The aroma of citrus was shown to bring neuroendocrine hormone levels back to normal in patients suffering from depression, so that their moods were elevated. This allows dosages of antidepressants to be reduced.[105] Hiba oil can also reduce depression,[106] and just three minutes of lavender oil aromatherapy can do the same.[107] Other oils with antidepressant-like effects are patchouli, sweet marjoram, jasmine, clary sage, cypress, lavandin, and ylang-ylang. Essential oils are also important in combating fatigue associated with depression. Lemon, pine, grapefruit, and eucalyptus oils can give a boost of energy. Using oils is a very safe and nonaddictive way to alleviate depression and boost energy without relying so heavily on antidepressant medications.

58. MEDITATION

Meditation began in Eastern cultures thousands of years ago as a way to achieve mental peace and tranquility. It is a state of thoughtless awareness in which the meditator is completely alert and can perform daily tasks with a calm and silent mind. When in this state, stress hormones are reduced in the body. This lowers blood pressure, heart rate, and blood glucose levels. Sleep is improved, the immune system responds better, and the risk of abdominal weight gain is reduced. And it is not necessary to sit quietly still in the lotus position to achieve a meditative state!

The process of achieving inner peace and quiet is unique for each individual. Some people prefer grounding oils to keep unnecessary thoughts away. Try sandalwood, patchouli, myrrh, vetiver, and spikenard. Others achieve this state by connecting with their spirituality and enhancing enlightenment. Frankincense, helichrysum, rosemary, myrtle, cinnamon leaf, and cypress are good choices for this. Adding natural sedatives to the mix like lavender, clary sage, chamomile, and ylang-ylang can also help achieve this relaxed state.

59. PASSION

Passion is an intoxicating pull toward someone or something that is greatly desired. There is physical passion between people and intellectual passion for knowledge, advancement, and servitude in careers or hobbies. The pursuit of passion leads to fulfillment, excitement, and bliss. It makes us feel like we are achieving our purpose in life. Everyday stress can suppress these feeling and cause passion to wane. This can be disappointing or frustrating. To rev up the enthusiasm again, use essential oils.

Blending variations of ginger, cinnamon leaf, clove, jasmine, vanilla, cardamom, patchouli, neroli, frankincense, myrrh, and angelica oils can help renew or elevate interests and desires. Place 3 drops of any of these oils in a diffuser and inhale for thirty minutes in the morning. If you are out at work or running errands, apply 3 drops of the mix to a teaspoon of jojoba oil and dab on the wrists, neck, temples, or back of the knees.

60. PATIENCE

At times, situations can arise or take unexpected turns that invoke negative feelings of anger, resentment, or annoyance. Working through these feelings without acting in a hostile manner requires patience. In an age when immediate gratification is the norm, acting with patience can be quite difficult for many and is a skill that needs to be honed. It takes time, but being kind to oneself, mindful of thoughts and actions, and aware of consequences can change the way we react to situations so that we approach them with thoughtfulness and accountability.

Inhaling the aroma of essential oils has a physiological effect on the limbic system of the brain and can alter moods and feelings. When patience is being tested, essential oils can dissipate anger, reduce anxiety, calm the mind, and provide clarity to a situation.

Add a drop each of bergamot, Roman chamomile, and lavender to a diffuser and inhale for thirty minutes. When on the go, dab a mixture on the wrists consisting of 1 drop each of ylang-ylang, sandalwood, and sweet orange essential oils to a teaspoon of sweet almond oil. Inhale when needed. Other oils to consider are patchouli, rosewood, geranium, vetiver, spruce, blue chamomile, sweet marjoram, and vanilla.

....

61. STRESS

Negative experiences cause us to react and respond to situations and people. This causes stress on the mind and body, even unknowingly. Stress can come from dangerous physical situations, work or home life, worry and tension, or fatigue. When stressed, the body releases chemicals into the blood that boost energy so we can manage the stressful times. The long-term effects of chronic stress can lead to weight gain, insomnia, anxiety, sexual dysfunction, and fatigue. The immune system functions suboptimally, increasing susceptibility to infections and disease.

One of the first steps to reduce stress is to relax. Deep breaths to fill the body with oxygen will help. Deep breathing with air diffused with aromatic essential oils is even better! Essential oils have the ability to alter mood and dissipate stress. Inhaling yuzu essential oil for ten minutes significantly decreased tension, anxiety, anger, and confusion in healthy women.[108] Lavender and fennel oils were also shown to reduce emotional stress.[109, 110] To ease physical and mental tension, take a warm shower and add several drops of essential oil to the shower floor. Cover the drain with a washcloth for a few minutes to prevent the oils from washing away. Inhale deeply. In addition to yuzu, lavender, and fennel essential oils, try rose, frankincense, Roman chamomile, bergamot, clove, vanilla, sweet basil, vetiver, ylang-ylang, or geranium.

CHAPTER 3

RECLAIMING BEAUTY

62. ACNE

Acne is a skin condition that results in pimples, blackheads, white-heads, cysts, nodules, and papules. It often appears on the face, but it can also show up on the neck, chest, back, upper arms, shoul-ders, and buttocks. Acne is the most common skin problem in the United States. It happens when dead skin cells stick together with sebum (oil) inside the pore. They become trapped. Bacteria living on the skin can sometimes get stuck in the pores with the dead skin cells. This provides a perfect breeding ground for them, and they quickly multiply. The skin becomes inflamed. If the acne goes deeper into the skin, a nodule or cyst forms. Typically, acne appears in teenagers and young adults, but it can affect anyone, even babies. Scars and dark spots on the skin can result. Mild acne can be treated with over-the-counter products that contain benzo-yl peroxide or salicylic acid. It takes four to eight weeks of using the product for acne to clear. For best resolution, a dermatologist should treat more severe cases. Prescription-grade topical treat-ments, whole body treatments like antibiotics, or office procedures involving lasers, lights, or chemicals may be used.

Rosemary essential oil has strong antibacterial properties. A study tested the effect of rosemary oil on *Propionibacterium acnes* (*P. acnes*), bacteria living in the follicles and pores of skin. They can grow in numbers and trigger inflammation, resulting in acne. Rosemary oil drastically impaired the bacteria by destroying the outer membranes and leaking their cytoplasmic contents. Cell death occurred in eight hours.[111] Add 3 drops of rosemary essential oil to a teaspoon of virgin coconut oil and apply directly on acne after washing the face. Coconut oil is effective at eliminating *P. acnes* as well, so this combination will clear the skin by destroying the bacteria that clog the pores with debris. Tea tree oil, lavender oil, oregano, bergamot, geranium, and frankincense can also be added to carrier oils and used for their antibacterial properties.

63. AGE SPOTS

Spending a lot of time outdoors is a healthy way to grow up, but all those years of sun exposure without sunscreen protection can cause the appearance of flat brown, grey, or black areas of pigmentation on the skin called age spots. They typically appear on the areas of the skin most exposed to the sun, like the face, hands, arms, chest, and shoulders. Ultraviolet radiation from the sun speeds up the production of melanin, creating a darker pigmentation of the skin known as a tan. After many years of sun exposure, melanin pigments can become clumped together, forming oval or round spots. These spots are generally harmless. Some people opt to treat them for cosmetic reasons. Prescription-strength creams containing retinol or hydroquinone are effective at fading the age spots. Microdermabrasion, laser treatments, chemical peels, and light therapy are also used.

Frankincense is the oil most used to fade age spots. It promotes skin healing, aids in the generation of new cells, deeply nourishes, and absorbs easily into the skin. Dilute 3 drops of frankincense essential oil in a teaspoon of jojoba oil and massage into the skin in a circular motion. After a few weeks, age spots should be noticeably lighter. Continue this practice twice daily. In a few months, the age spots should be significantly less noticeable or completely gone. Carrot seed, geranium, and lemon essential oils are also used to fade age spots. Use in the same manner as frankincense oil.

. . . .

64. BRUISES

Often, bruises happen from events that go unnoticed, such as bumping into a railing or catching a hip on the kitchen counter. Others happen from vigorous exercise, bleeding disorders, or blood-thinning medications. Elderly persons are more susceptible to bruises because they have thinner skin that gives less support to the blood vessels underneath. When the skin in injured, the blood cells under the skin are damaged. They leak blood, which pools underneath the surface of the skin, giving rise to a tender and sometimes painful black or blue mark. The bruise begins to heal and turns yellow or green. It eventually fades as the blood is reabsorbed. Ice and, later, heat can be applied to the bruise to reduce swelling and improve circulation to the area.

When a bruise develops on the skin, apply a cold compress to the area to ease swelling and to constrict the capillaries at the surface of the skin. This reduces the amount of blood released from them. After blood flow has stopped and the bruised area is defined, prepare 1 teaspoon of arnica lotion combined with 2 drops of essential oils known for their anti-inflammatory and pain-reducing properties. Helichrysum, lavender, chamomile, rosemary, and lemongrass oils are recommended. Add a third drop of yarrow, cinnamon leaf, or parsley oil to improve circulation and promote the body's natural healing process. Swelling should further reduce, along with any tenderness, pain, and discoloration.

65. CELLULITE

Normal fat beneath the skin can push against connective tissue and cause the skin above it to pucker. This results in a dimpled appearance of the skin that many find undesirable. It is extremely common in women and occurs most often on the hips, thighs, buttocks, and stomach. This is not just a condition for overweight people, because thin individuals can have cellulite too. There is a strong genetic link, so if one generation had it, the next generation is likely to as well. To reduce the appearance of cellulite, stay hydrated, lose weight if needed, and exercise to tone the muscles and boost circulation to the areas.

Grapefruit essential oil is used to reduce water retention and swelling, both of which decrease the appearance of cellulite and eliminate toxins. Lemongrass, cedarwood, juniper berry, cypress, and sweet fennel oils reduce fluid retention too, but they also improve circulation. This brings more oxygen to the fat cells underneath the skin and helps the body remove toxic buildup. The result is smaller cells and less visible cellulite. To firm and tone the skin, use ginger, grapefruit, rosemary, and carrot seed essential oils. These will minimize the effects of fatty cells bulging to the surface. Make sure to dilute these oils in a carrier oil before massaging into the skin.

66. CHAPPED LIPS

Chapped lips are characterized by dry, cracked lips that can be red and itchy. The skin on the lips is very thin and provides only a small measure of protection to the tissue underneath. It does not contain any sebaceous glands to produce moisturizing oil, and water loss from the lips is much higher than anywhere else on the body. Other exacerbating factors include dry environmental conditions, lip licking, sun damage, vitamin deficiencies, medication, and infections. It's easy to see why chapped lips are such a common problem for many.

The first step to achieving smooth, soft lips is to exfoliate with a gentle lip scrub. To make your own at home, combine 2 teaspoons of white sugar, 1/2 teaspoon of jojoba oil, 1 teaspoon of honey, and 1 drop of peppermint essential oil. Mix in a small glass jar and keep in the bathroom. Use daily or when lips are chapped. It's also important to moisturize the lips and keep them hydrated throughout the day. Add 1 tablespoon of fractionated coconut oil, 3 drops of lavender oil, and 3 drops of frankincense oil to a glass roller bottle. Shake and apply to the lips as needed throughout the day. These oils will keep a protective layer over the lips and prevent moisture loss, rapidly heal dry skin, and increase its strength and elasticity. Rosewood, jasmine, geranium, patchouli, and sandalwood oils can be substituted in these recipes.

67. CRACKED HEELS

The skin on the heels of the feet can become dry and crack. The tissue around the rim of the heels may thicken, causing calluses. Cracks can occur in the thick calluses, too, especially if there is too much weight bearing down on the fat pads under the heels in the absence of shoe support. Prolonged standing and improper footwear can increase pressure on the heels, forcing them to expand sideways. If the skin is dry, this increased pressure will cause the skin to crack. Some medical or skin conditions can dry the skin, leading to this problem. Most cases of cracked heels are just irritating, but if the condition is severe, it may become painful and unsightly.

It's important to wear proper footwear to support the foot and alleviate excessive pressure on the heels. Shoes with thick soles and closed backs are recommended. To repair the heels, begin by debriding the callused tissue to reduce its thickness; some cracks won't heal if this extra, tough skin is not removed. Then soak the feet in a warm footbath with several drops of Roman chamomile, sandalwood, and jasmine. This should soften the skin and bring moisture to the heels. After 5 minutes, remove the feet from the bath and pat dry. Using a pumice stone, gently exfoliate the dry, tough skin on the heels. Rinse the feet and pat dry again. Apply an ointment of 1 tablespoon sweet almond oil, 2 drops rose essential oil, and 1 drop cedarwood essential oil. Exfoliate every other day, but apply the ointment every morning and evening. Alternate oils to use are rosewood, geranium, mandarin, lavender, and patchouli.

68. DANDRUFF

Dandruff is a chronic condition marked by the flaking of skin cells on the scalp. They are visible as white, oily-looking flakes of skin in the hair and on the shoulders. It is not a dangerous condition, but it can be embarrassing for some people. Dandruff is usually worse in the fall and winter when the scalp is subjected to the drier, cooler outdoor air and heated indoor air, which depletes moisture in the skin. It can be caused by not shampooing enough so that dead skin cells mix with oils. This causes a buildup and subsequent shedding of these cells as dandruff.

Yeast on the scalp can irritate the skin of some people and cause an overproduction of skin cells, which will flake off as dandruff. Dry skin can cause smaller, drier flakes to appear. One of the most common causes of dandruff, however, is seborrheic dermatitis. This is a condition in which oily skin is covered in flaky white or yellow scales. Mild cases are easy to treat with daily cleansing to reduce oil and skin cell buildup. Other cases are more difficult and may need medicated shampoos. Some shampoos contain antifungal and antibacterial agents to kill the microbes. Others work by slowing the death rate of skin cells to reduce buildup and flaking.

If the source of dandruff is the yeast-causing seborrheic dermatitis, then using tea tree oil will help reduce the overproduction of skin cells. A 5 percent tea tree oil shampoo significantly lessened the severity of dandruff, itchiness of the scalp, and greasiness of the hair in patients with dandruff compared to patients using a placebo shampoo.[112] It appears that tea tree oil doesn't have to be very concentrated to be effective. Another study found that at just

0.5 percent, tea tree oil destroyed the yeast responsible for causing dandruff.[113] The antifungal and anti-inflammatory properties of this oil safely, speedily, and effectively destroy the pathogens causing dandruff and attenuate the distressing symptoms associated with it by reducing redness, itch, and irritation of the scalp.

If dry skin is the culprit, lavender, thyme, peppermint, rosemary, geranium, myrrh, jasmine, and patchouli essential oils can be used to moisturize, calm, and soothe inflamed skin and increase circulation to the scalp. To get rid of dandruff, make a solution of 1/2 cup of apple cider vinegar, 35 drops of tea tree oil, and 25 drops of jasmine oil. After shampooing, take approximately 2 to 3 tablespoons of the solution and massage it into the scalp. Let it sit for a few minutes and then rinse it out with warm water. Use three times a week until dandruff is gone.

69. DEODoRANT

Sweating is a natural function of the body used to reduce body heat. Sweat itself is odorless. The warm, moist environment, however, is a breeding ground for bacteria, and they thrive in the armpit in these conditions. The bacteria break down keratin protein on the surface of the skin and produce odor-causing fatty acids and ammonia. To reduce armpit odor, wash regularly and keep the armpit dry. Most people use antiperspirants to reduce sweating or deodorants to mask odor.

Because sweating is a natural process to regulate body temperature and remove toxins from the body, allowing the body to sweat is recommended. Deodorants can help mask odor for a period of time, but bacteria can overpower even the most pungent scents.

HEALTH

WELL-BEING

BEAUTY

HOME

The best way to be odor-free is to make sure the bacteria don't have a chance to grow in the armpits. Antibacterial essential oils should keep away any offending odors. Mix 1/4 cup of jojoba oil with 36 drops of any of the following oils, based on personal aromatic preference: lavender, lemongrass, cinnamon leaf, tea tree, clove, eucalyptus, peppermint, bergamot, oregano, thyme, basil, rosemary, ginger, sandalwood, lemon, and patchouli. Massage into a clean armpit. The jojoba oil will absorb into the skin without leaving a greasy or wet feeling. As the day wears on, reapply as needed.

70. FRESH BREATH

No one wants bad breath, but everyone gets it now and then. Some foods, like onions and garlic, are common culprits for bad breath, and their strong odors linger until the food has been digested by the body. Poor dental hygiene is another source of bad breath. Food particles that remain in the mouth become food for bacteria, which grow and thrive, emitting foul-smelling toxins into the mouth. Yeast infections, cavities, smoking, dry mouth, and some diseases are other causes. Using mouthwash as part of an oral hygiene regimen is optional, but many choose to include it. Most mouthwashes are antiseptic and are used to decrease the microbes in the mouth to prevent cavities, gingivitis, and bad breath. Others are advertised as reducing inflammation, pain, or dry mouth caused by infection or disease. About 20 milliliters of mouthwash is gargled for thirty seconds or more then spit out.

If bad breath is a problem, using diluted antibacterial essential oils as a mouthwash can remove the bacteria from the mouth and stop their metabolic byproducts from emitting offensive odors. Black sage essential oil inhibited the growth of *P. gingivalis*, an oral bacteria that contributes to gum disease.[114] Other antibacterial oils to use are clove, peppermint, oregano, orange, cinnamon leaf, and lavender.

Essential oils can also be used to eliminate *Candida* yeast infections in the mouth that cause bad breath. Lavender essential oil inhibits the growth of both the yeast and hyphal forms of *C. albicans*.[115] The compounds eugenol and thymus have also been shown to have anti-*Candida* activity.[116] These are found in clove, cinnamon, nutmeg, geranium, oregano, basil, vanilla, dill, lemon balm, bergamot, oregano, and thyme essential oils.

In addition to brushing twice a day and flossing once a day, use essential oils as an oral rinse to eliminate bacteria or fungi in the mouth. Two drops of peppermint oil or clove oil can be combined with a teaspoon of virgin coconut oil—which is also great for destroying bacteria in the mouth—and swished around the mouth for a minute before spitting out in the garbage. Do this once a day. Choose the oil depending on the source of bad breath.

71. HAIR CONDITIONER

There are about one hundred thousand to one hundred fifty thousand hairs on the human head. Those are a lot of strands to take care of! Each strand of hair consists of three layers, with the outer layer, or cuticle, protecting the inner two layers. When the hair is healthy, the scales of the cuticle overlap tightly and protect the inner layers. When it becomes damaged, however, the scales of the

HEALTH

WELL-BEING

BEAUTY

HOME

cuticle loosen and separate, exposing the layers underneath. The hair looks dry and dull and may break easily. The inner layers can become damaged from exposure to the UV rays of the sun, heat, pollution, chlorine, or any of the array of chemicals found in hair products and treatments.

Essential oils can be used to create shiny, soft, strong hair that looks smooth and healthy. Many of these oils are antioxidants that will protect newly conditioned hair from future damage and lock in moisture for long-term manageability. Mix 9 drops of essential oils in 1 tablespoon of sweet almond oil, and massage into wet hair. If hair is longer, double the recipe. For normal hair, choose sweet orange, rosemary, or eucalyptus essential oils. Basil, cedarwood, lemon, and bergamot oils work well with oily hair, and dry hair likes lavender, ylang-ylang, geranium, frankincense, rosemary, and sandalwood oils. Let the solution sit on the hair for twenty minutes, then rinse and shampoo. No other conditioner is needed.

72. HAIR LOSS

Hair grows everywhere on the body except the palms of the hands and the soles of the feet. Countless hours and money are spent trying to get rid of hair on the body, yet every hair on the head is clung to as if it were made of gold. Healthy, shiny, lustrous hair is a sign of beauty and a point of fashion and personal expression. Hair loss is common in men and can even happen in women and children. As excessive hair falls out and bald spots appear, a person may undergo significant anxiety and feel exposed, inadequate, or unattractive. It happens when hair follicles on the head no longer produce new hair cells. Heredity plays a large role in hair loss and affects the age it begins, the rate at which it occurs, and the pattern it takes. Medications, disease, and hormone changes may also cause excessive hair loss. To counteract hair loss, people use medications to try to stimulate growth or slow loss. Others undergo surgery and transplant tiny plugs of skin-containing hairs into the scalp. These come with side effects like rapid heart rate, sexual dysfunction, pain, infection, and scarring.

Thyme, rosemary, lavender, and cedarwood were investigated for their role in hair growth. After seven months of treatment, patients who massaged these diluted essential oils into their scalp each day saw significant improvement in hair regrowth compared to patients who massaged their scalps with only carrier oils.[117] Lavender oil on its own proved to promote hair regrowth as well. The backs of mice treated with lavender oil saw a significant increase in the number and depth of follicles as well as an increase in the thickness of the dermal layer in which the follicles sit.[118]

Oils that increase circulation can also stimulate hair growth by bringing more blood and nutrients to the cells on the scalp to keep them functioning, dividing, and growing. Areas of the scalp that are patchy from hair loss can begin to grow hair once again. To grow hair, mix 3 drops each of lavender, cedarwood, and thyme essential oils in 1 tablespoon of jojoba oil. Apply to the scalp and let the oils absorb into the skin. Do this daily to see results. Other oils to use are ylang-ylang, palmarosa, cypress, sandalwood, black pepper, clove, lemon, and rosewood.

73. MOISTURIZE FACIAL SKIN

Having hydrated and moisturized skin gives a healthy glow and a more youthful appearance. Dehydration causes skin cells to build up on the surface, rather than slough off, resulting in a dry, rough appearance. Elasticity is lost, and the skin becomes tight and possibly cracked. Fine lines and wrinkles are more pronounced. Moisture loss can be a result of sun damage, hot showers, wind, excessive consumption of diuretic drinks, avoidance of moisturizers, or harsh skin products. It worsens with age due to the decline in oil gland activity and the lowered ability of the skin to hold onto water.

Rehydrating the top layers of skin and locking in moisture will help improve the appearance and feel of dry skin. The most effective products that do this attract and seal in moisture and smooth the skin by filling in the spaces between the skin cells. Before applying a moisturizer, always wash the face first to prevent sealing in dirt and debris. Failure to do so may result in clogged pores. To make a light, aromatic, and nourishing facial serum to banish dry skin, use oils like rose, palmarosa, German chamomile, myrrh, frankincense, lavender, clary sage, sandalwood, geranium, and neroli. This can be made by combining 1/3 cup argan oil, 3 tablespoons of rosehip seed oil, and 20 to 28 drops of your favorite essential oil (or oils). Store in a dark glass bottle and shake before each use.

74. NAIL FUNGUS

Fungal infections are extremely common and can infect any part of the body. When fungi target the fingernails or toenails, white or yellow spots may begin to appear. These spots then merge to form patches and spread out. The nails become thicker, brittle, or discolored, and the edges start to crumble. The symptoms occur slowly and may eventually result in the nail detaching from the skin and falling off.

Fungal infections can actually be a sign of candida overgrowth in the body. *Candida albicans* is a very common fungus in humans and can grow out of control in people with weakened or compromised immune systems. The good bacteria in the gut cannot compete with *Candida*, and a systemic invasion may begin which can show up as a fungal infection of the nails. Over-the-counter treatments are available, but they are not always effective, and the chance of reoccurrence is high. Prescribed oral antifungal drugs can be used that allow new growth of the nail to be fungi-free. This is a slow process and may cause a variety of side effects from a skin rash to liver disease. Medicated polishes and creams are used, but these can take a year to get rid of the fungi. The nail can also be surgically removed, but it grows back slowly.

There are many essential oils that have antifungal properties. Oregano, thyme, rosemary, pine, chamomile, frankincense, lemongrass, cinnamon leaf, clove, lavender, and tea tree essential oils are some of them. Lavender oil was tested against fifty-one strains of *Candida albicans* in a laboratory setting and effectively inhibited fungal growth and the spread of infection.[119] Tea tree oil demonstrated the same activity against thirty-two strains of *C. albicans.*[120] These essential oils can be used singly or in combination to topically treat fungal nail infections. Simply mix 3 drops of oregano (or other) essential oil in a teaspoon of apricot kernel oil. Dip a cotton ball in the oil and rub it over and around the nails. Let the oil soak in. Repeat morning and night until the infected nail grows out and is replaced by a healthy nail.

75. NAIL STRENGTHENER

Nails can become either brittle and dry due to moisture loss or soft and brittle due to too much moisture. Sometimes, disease or diet is the culprit, but more often, external factors are responsible. This is particularly true if the toenails are strong but the fingernails are weak. The constant wetting and drying of the nails through numerous hand washings, dish washings, showers, and chores—not to mention the use of detergents, harsh cleaners, and nail polish removers—all wreak havoc on nail health and can cause irreversible damage. Often, the damaged nails have to be grown out. As the new nails grow in, take care to make sure they remain healthy. Wear gloves when doing chores, moisturize the cuticles, soak the nails in oil, and clip or file them regularly.

Add 10 drops of essential oils to a tablespoon of grapeseed oil. Grapeseed oil is light, non-greasy, and very moisturizing. It's loaded with antioxidants and is a wonderful source of vitamin E that will nourish the nails. Essential oils like lavender, rosemary, lemon, cypress, geranium, and grapefruit can help retain moisture and reduce brittleness, flaking, and splitting. Apply the serum each night to the nails and cuticles and massage for one minute.

76. OILY HAIR

The scalp contains sebaceous glands that produce oil. This oil keeps the hair healthy, moisturized, smooth, and strong. The amount of oil that is produced can change with the seasons, the climate, stress, product use, or hormones. Sometimes, too much oil is produced and causes the hair to look stringy and greasy. Wash the hair each day, if needed. Use shampoos that do not contain sulfate extracts. They cause sebaceous glands to become overly activated. Try to wash hair in the morning, because the sebaceous glands are particularly active at night and secrete more oil during this time. Go easy on the conditioner and use lukewarm water, not hot.

Some oils like rosemary, lavender, lemongrass, and chamomile are thought to normalize oil production and can be useful in calming overactive sebaceous glands in the scalp. Combine 6 drops of rosemary essential oil with a tablespoon of melted virgin coconut oil and massage into the wet scalp. Leave on for 30 minutes, then wash out with a mild shampoo. Other essential oils to consider for oily hair are lemon, cypress, bergamot, eucalyptus, and juniper berry oils.

77. PERFUME

The pleasing aroma of essential oils mixed with other ingredients creates a limitless variety of perfumes that are used to scent people, pets, creams, lotions, gels, candles, and living spaces. Really, an object can be infused with perfume to make it more appealing

HEALTH

WELL-BEING

BEAUTY

HOME

to a particular gender or demographic. There are different types of perfumes, depending on the concentration of aromatic essential oils in the final product. Perfume typically contains 20 percent aromatic compounds, eau de perfume has about 15 percent, eau de toilette, about 10 percent, and cologne, 5 percent. The higher the concentration of aromatic compounds, the more intense and longer lasting the scent. In addition to varying concentrations of essential oils, these products contain many other ingredients, both natural and synthetic. Some of these trigger asthma reactions, nausea, headaches, increased skin sensitivity to ultraviolet radiation, or allergic skin reactions. Most companies keep their ingredients proprietary, so the consumer is not aware of what they are putting on their body. Long-term use of perfumes may have health consequences that have yet to be uncovered.

Essential oils are the basis of perfumes, so why not simply use essential oils diluted in a carrier oil as perfume? The desired scent can be uniquely selected, depending on the wearer's mood. Essential oils are volatile and evaporate quickly, but the carrier oil will keep the essential oil in solution much longer. When the aroma does eventually die off, more can be applied, if desired. Both liquid and solid perfumes can be made at home. For a solid perfume, melt a tablespoon of grated beeswax on the stove. Once almost melted, mix in a tablespoon of carrier oil. Camellia seed oil, fractionated coconut oil, and sweet almond oil are some good choices. Stir until the beeswax and carrier oil are fully combined. Remove from the stove and immediately stir in about 60 drops of essential oils. Choose your blend beforehand and have it ready to go; this mixture sets quickly. Pour into a glass or ceramic container with a lid. It should set in about ten minutes and be ready to wear.

78. SCARS

A thickened and permanent patch of skin that forms over a wound when the skin is injured by a cut, scrape, sore, acne, or burn is a scar. Scars will fade over time, but they never go away. Some scars are small and not bothersome to the person. Others are larger or in conspicuous places like the face. These can make a person feel self-conscious or that it negatively impacts their physical attractiveness. There are a number of procedures to reduce the appearance of scars. Chemical peel, dermabrasion, and laser therapy are a few. These require trips to the doctor and can be expensive. They also come with a risk of side effects including infection, redness, pain, and bruising.

There are different types of scars, but one kind, called a hypertrophic scar, is characterized by a raised appearance. This is due to excessive tissue developing over the wound during healing. Surgical removal of the excess tissue and steroid hormones have been used to treat these scars, but they come with complications. Chinese lovage essential oil was used as an alternative in a study on formed hypertrophic scars in rabbit ears. The essential oil was applied once a day for twenty-eight days, resulting in significant improvements in the appearance of the scars.[121] Chinese lovage essential oil may be effective in shrinking these scars and making them less visible. Marigold essential oil is good for reducing the appearance of acne scars. Frankincense, myrrh, rose, helichrysum, cedarwood, lemon, geranium, lavender, carrot seed, and patchouli oils can also be used for any scar type. Fresh scars respond better to treatment than old scars, so promptly use these oils when the scar

HEALTH

WELL-BEING

BEAUTY

HOME

is new. To create a treatment serum, mix 2 tablespoons of sweet almond oil and 2 drops each of lavender, patchouli, and helichrysum essential oils. Apply two to three times a day.

79. SHAMPOO

Shampoo is a cleansing product for hair to remove dirt and oil. There are shampoos designed for color-treated hair, dandruff, limp hair, overprocessed hair, dry hair, oily hair, and so on. Many shampoos leave product buildup on the hair and strip the oils without adding back moisture. This causes the hair to become dry, brittle, and frizzy. The majority of shampoos have a long list of chemicals to create lather, rinse easily, smell good, and feel luxurious. Many of these compounds have been found to be irritants and allergens and have health consequences—not only on the person using the shampoo but on the environment as the shampoo gets washed down the drain.

Some essential oils are moisturizing, while others are great for reducing oil production. All oils smell wonderful and make the hair amazingly fragrant. Use them in homemade shampoos to impart their powerful effects and to cleanse the hair in a safe, nontoxic way. Shampoo is very easy to make and allows the user to customize the ingredients to their taste and particular hair issues. A base recipe that can be used for all shampoos is 1/2 cup coconut milk and 1/2 cup liquid castile soap. If the coconut milk doesn't contain guar gum, then add 1/4 teaspoon of xanthan gum to the recipe as a thickener.

Now here comes the fun part! For dry hair, add 1/2 teaspoon of a carrier oil like sweet almond, safflower, or grapeseed oil.

Experiment to see what works best for you. Then add 20 drops of essential oils. Some great ones to choose from for dry hair are palmarosa, rosemary, clary sage, lavender, myrrh, peppermint, spearmint, geranium, and sandalwood.

For oily hair, skip the carrier oil and add 20 drops of any of these oils: basil, cedarwood, clary sage, patchouli, tea tree, lavender, lime, rosemary, eucalyptus, and cypress.

Normal hair doesn't need the carrier oil, either, but will benefit from clary sage, lavender, rosemary, cedarwood, geranium, and sweet orange essential oils. Put all the ingredients in an old shampoo bottle and shake vigorously to mix. Before each use, shake the bottle to mix any ingredients that have settled. The antimicrobial activity of the essential oils will keep this shampoo good for two to three weeks.

80. SUNSCREEN

Excessive exposure to the sun can cause sunburn, promote the development of wrinkles and sagging skin, and increase the risk of melanoma and squamous cell carcinoma. It is important to receive some sun so that the skin can make vitamin D, which is essential for bone growth and remodeling, immune function, and neuromuscular activity. Just as important, however, is to protect the skin from the harmful ultraviolet rays of the sun. Sunscreens do just this. They come as lotions, sprays, gels, and sticks and are applied topically. They either absorb the ultraviolet rays or reflect sunlight. Many sunscreens block only ultraviolet B sunlight, which causes sunburns, while ultraviolet A sunlight increases skin damage and the risk of skin cancers. Broad-spectrum sunscreens will block both types of rays. Some of the ingredients used in commercially available sunscreens include PABA, phenylbenzimidazole sulfonic acid, sulisobenzone, and octocrylene (among many others) that can irritate the skin and increase damaging reactive oxygen species and DNA defects.

Some essential oils are natural sunscreens that have an SPF (sun protection factor) between 1 and 7.[122] For an SPF of 7, that means a seventh of the sun's ultraviolet B radiation reaches the skin. It blocks only ultraviolet B rays, meaning it will help prevent the skin from burning but doesn't provide protection against ultraviolet A rays, which increase the risk of cancer and photodermatitis. Peppermint and tulsi essential oils have an SPF of around 7, while lavender and lemongrass essential oils have an SPF of around 6. Eucalyptus, tea tree, and rose essential oils have lower SPFs, between 1 and 3.[123] Adding peppermint oil to a carrier oil like olive oil (SPF 8) or coconut oil (SPF 7) makes a natural, safe, and moisturizing sunscreen when spending small amounts of time in the sun. If extended periods are to be spent outdoors, reapply frequently and consider supplementing with a product that supplies ultraviolet A protection as well. A mixture of 1/4 cup coconut oil, 1/4 cup shea butter, 2 tablespoons zinc oxide, 1 teaspoon vitamin E oil, 50 drops of peppermint oil, and 25 drops of lavender oil is another option.

81. STRETCH MARKS

Stretch marks can develop during periods of intense growth, like puberty or pregnancy, or amid rapid weight changes. The middle layers of skin are stretched beyond their elastic capacity and tear.

This can also happen when medical conditions cause elevated levels of cortisone to be released from the adrenal glands, resulting in the skin losing suppleness. Products with corticosteroids can also render this effect. Scar tissue forms as narrow reddish-purple lines, which eventually fade to silvery white. Stretch marks are extremely common and occur most often on the stomach, thighs, hips, buttocks, upper arms, and lower back. Some stretch marks disappear over time, but others remain throughout life. To minimize the appearance of stretch marks, medicated lotions, microdermabrasion, and laser therapy are sometimes used. These don't guarantee results, however, and can be expensive.

A natural alternative to heal the skin, restore elasticity, and make stretch marks disappear is to use essential oils. Helichrysum, rosehip, and patchouli are useful in generating new skin cells by increasing cell turnover. Lavender, neroli, and frankincense rejuvenate and revitalize skin and start the healing process. Geranium and jasmine improve the skin's elasticity.

To make a cream to use at home, combine 1/2 cup of shea butter with 10 drops of lavender and 10 drops of frankincense essential oils. Apply morning and night to the stretch marks.

82. SUNBURN

Sitting outside in the sun for too long without the protection of sunscreen can cause the skin to burn. The ultraviolet rays of the sun penetrate the skin and increase the rate of melanin production. This is the body's way of protecting the skin from the damaging effects of the sun, but when exposure is too long or the rays too intense,

HEALTH

WELL-BEING

BEAUTY

HOME

melanin is not enough and the skin burns. It becomes red, painful, and swollen. It is hot to the touch and may form small fluid-filled blisters. Tanning lamps can burn the skin in the same way the sun does. Even the sun's rays that have been reflected off the surface of water, sand, ice, and snow can give a sunburn. Cloudy days emit 80 percent of the sun's ultraviolet rays, so caution is needed for outdoor activities on these days as well. Sunburned skin begins to heal itself within a few days. Pain relievers and corticosteroids are often used for pain and to control itching.

While nothing but time can be used to remove a sunburn, the symptoms can be managed with essential oils. Anti-inflammatory, antibacterial, and pain-reducing essential oils like lavender, frankincense, peppermint, ginger, rosemary, and eucalyptus can help prevent an infection from invading the wounded skin, reduce swelling, and take the sting out of even the softest touch. Other ones to use include Roman chamomile, sandalwood, manuka, and geranium. Take a bath in cool water with 1/2 cup apple cider vinegar and sprinkle in a few drops of lavender oil. This will speed healing time and increase comfort by reducing itching and pain. Another way to soothe the skin is to gently massage a mixture of 1 teaspoon of aloe vera gel with 1 drop of peppermint oil, 1 drop of Roman chamomile oil, and 1 drop of lavender oil. This will cool the skin and provide itch and pain relief.

83. TEETH WHITENER

Bright, white teeth make for a beautiful smile and give a younger and healthier appearance. There are many products in stores that claim to whiten teeth. Whitening toothpastes remove surface stains with mild abrasive agents and can achieve about one shade of difference. Whitening gels, strips, and trays contain hydrogen peroxide or other bleaching agents, which lighten deep within the tooth. Results usually last about four months. Some mouthwashes contain ingredients to whiten teeth, but they are less effective and results are often not seen for twelve weeks. Dentists can also dramatically whiten teeth in their offices in one visit. Tooth sensitivity and tissue irritation are a few side effects of the bleaching process.

Bacteria in the mouth build up a biofilm on the teeth called plaque. Plaque can cause the teeth to become discolored and look yellow. Peppermint, sage, and Australian tea tree oils are potent in reducing oral bacteria.[124] Peppermint and sage can be used as an oral rinse to eliminate the bacteria responsible for discoloring teeth and maintain a brighter smile. Tea tree oil should not be used in case some is accidentally swallowed; it can be toxic if ingested. Combine a mashed-up strawberry with a teaspoon of virgin coconut oil. Mix to form a paste. Add 3 drops of peppermint essential oil and combine. Brush the teeth with this mixture for two minutes. Spit into the garbage and rinse the mouth. Brush as normal with toothpaste.

84. TOOTHPASTE

Toothpastes are gels, pastes, or powders that are used with a toothbrush to clean the teeth. They help remove food debris and bacteria, which prevents the formation of plaque and tartar that can lead to tooth decay and gum disease. Most commercial toothpastes contain a variety of chemicals including detergents, mild abrasives, binding agents, fluoride, and flavor to ensure that the toothpaste foams well, tastes good, removes surface stains, and strengthens teeth. Some have special additives to improve whitening power, sensitivity, and tartar control. Not all these ingredients are safe, and some have been known to cause canker sores or disrupt hormones. Others are potential carcinogens or even considered lethal (fluoride) if swallowed in acute doses.

Natural toothpastes can be purchased online or in stores, but not all these are as healthy as they pretend to be. The movement to make products at home using all natural ingredients is on the rise. Homemade toothpaste is easy to make, costs little, and cleans and whitens the teeth just as well as commercial toothpastes. Before buying your next tube of toothpaste, consider making this recipe instead. Slowly melt 1/2 cup of virgin coconut oil in a glass jar placed in a pan of warm water on the stove. Once melted, add 2 tablespoons of baking soda and stir until combined. Next, mix in 1 tablespoon of powdered xylitol and 15 drops of essential oils. Stir well and allow the mixture to solidify. The toothpaste is now ready to use. Some essential oils to consider for their antibacterial properties are peppermint, spearmint, cinnamon leaf, clove, sage, and myrrh.

85. WRINKLES

The process of getting older involves many changes in the body. Arteries stiffen, bones lose density, memory declines, skin thins, and wrinkles appear. The rate at which these processes take place varies from person to person. Genetics and illness play a role in when and how we age, but our diet and lifestyle significantly impact the process. There are many theories of aging, but the free radical theory is growing in popularity as an explanation. It is thought that free radicals are responsible for age-related damage of cells and tissues. Free radicals are unstable molecules actively looking for an electron. They attack the nearest stable molecule and steal one of their electrons, making that molecule a free radical as well. This begins a chain reaction of creating free radicals that ultimately can destroy the cell.

The key to stopping these free radicals lies in the presence of antioxidants. Many essential oils contain antioxidant compounds, which donate electrons to make the free radicals stable. They no longer wreak havoc on cells and tissues, causing damage. The aging process is slowed. This happens throughout the body from the liver to the skin. Some of the best oils to use for their antioxidant properties are clove, myrrh, coriander, sweet fennel, clary sage, Roman chamomile, rose, marjoram, ylang-ylang, wintergreen, geranium, ginger, eucalyptus, cumin, and vetiver. Other oils are known for their ability to tighten and tone the skin. These include geranium, sandalwood, and frankincense. Frankincense also minimizes the appearance of age spots. Lavender and carrot seed oils regenerate the skin, while rose oil improves its elasticity. Each evening, mix a teaspoon of jojoba oil with 1 drop each of rose, frankincense, and Roman chamomile essential oils. Massage over the face and neck. Any remaining oil can be applied to the hands and chest.

HEALTH

WELL-BEING

BEAUTY

HOME

CHAPTER 4

RECONDITIONING YOUR HOME

HEALTH

WELL-BEING

BEAUTY

HOME

PEST CONTROL

86. BACTERIA ON DISH SPONGES

The kitchen is the place in the home that we want to keep the cleanest. After all, this is where food is prepared and eaten. We do our best to keep all manner of pests out of the kitchen, and the sight of one cockroach or fruit fly larvae crawling in the sink can have us running for the hills. Imagine, then, if you knew that scrubbing down countertops and washing glasses with a dish sponge may be spreading millions of bacteria all over everything it touches. Each sponge contains about ten million bacteria per square inch, some innocuous and some harmful. To ensure the health and safety of your family, sponges should be washed at temperatures above 180 degrees Fahrenheit and disinfected regularly.

Cleaning sponges with warm soap and water will get rid of surface dirt and some bacteria, but there are still many germs lurking behind, just waiting to multiply again. It's also really hard to rinse soap completely out of the sponge. There are some essential oils that have excellent antibacterial properties that can be used to destroy a variety of bacteria and keep sponges clean and disinfected. A study on the antibacterial activity of a number of essential oils against twenty-five genera of bacteria found that thyme, cinnamon leaf, bay, clove, bitter almond, Chinese lovage, pimento, marjoram, angelica, and nutmeg were the strongest at inhibiting bacterial growth and survival. Angelica oil was able to inhibit all twenty-five bacteria genera tested, followed by bay, cinnamon leaf, clove, and thyme oils.[125] Each evening, squeeze excess water out of the sponge. Spray all sides with a solution of 1/4 cup water, 1 teaspoon of castile soap, 10 drops of thyme oil, 10 drops of cinnamon leaf oil, and 5 drops of angelica oil. Just a few spritzes per side are needed. Squeeze the sponge to distribute the oils to the interior.

87. FLEAS ON DOGS

Fleas are small, copper-colored pests that live in warm, humid environments and feed on blood. They have strong hind legs and can jump onto pets from anywhere they can be found, whether it's other animals or from the environment. Fleas don't like light, so look on pets' bellies, hind legs, or deep within their fur to detect them. Small, pepper-like flakes are telltale signs of a flea infestation. These are the feces from the flea. Fleas live for several weeks on dogs and lay hundreds of eggs. The eggs can fall off pets and land on carpets, on furniture, on drapes, or even in floor cracks. They develop into larvae and feed on organic matter. As adults, they hop onto the nearest host. The bite of the flea causes itching in pets, and if the animal is allergic to the saliva of the flea, then skin infections, inflammation, and hair loss can result. Prescription pills or medicated shampoos can rid dogs of fleas. Some dishwashing liquid is commonly used as well.

HEALTH

WELL-BEING

BEAUTY

HOME

Essential oils can be used on dogs to exterminate fleas. Lemongrass, lavender, cedarwood, manuka, patchouli, eucalyptus, spearmint, and thyme are good ones to use. Because animals' sense of smell is heightened over humans, they may not like certain aromas. Apply a diluted oil to your hands, allow the animal to smell it, and see how they react. If they are turned off, try another one. If they don't appear to be bothered by the scent, you have a winner. Combine 1 to 3 drops of essential oils with 1/2 cup of dog shampoo. (Blue dish detergent works very well too.) Shampoo the dog, taking care to avoid the eyes. Once clear of fleas, make a deterrent spray using 5 drops of cedarwood oil, 2 drops of eucalyptus oil, and 2 drops of lavender oil in 1 cup of water.

As a word of caution, be very careful using essential oils around cats. They lack an important enzyme that breaks down and eliminates compounds that have been ingested, absorbed, or inhaled. Many essential oils can become toxic to cats, so it's best to avoid them unless they've been proven specifically safe for felines.

88. FOOD-SPOILING FUNGI

Fungi, specifically molds and yeasts, live in and on food. They secrete enzymes that break down the food so that they can absorb the nutrients. This is how they grow and thrive. The result is food that is off flavor, discolored, rotted, or contaminated with harmful mycotoxins. Fruits, vegetables, meats, breads, and sauces—just about any food sitting on the counter or in the fridge—are susceptible. There are a few foods that have built-in defenses that can ward off spoilage for long periods of time, but eventually, fungi will grow on them too (except honey). Companies in the food industry use chemical sprays to preserve foods and delay spoilage. Seeds and produce often get a dose of pesticides during the growing phases and another during transportation from the field to the store.

Buying organic food cuts down on pesticide use and reduces the chemical burden to the body. Organic food does spoil faster, however. Essential oils can be used to extend the shelf life of food, destroy potentially harmful fungi, and reduce the amounts of harmful toxins ingested. Eggplants with grey mold rot were treated with oregano essential oil, which was found to inhibit fungal growth without affecting fruit quality.[126] Allspice, cinnamon, clove, garlic, onion, oregano, savory, and thyme showed potent inhibitory effects on the growth of thirteen food-spoilage and industrial fungi,[127] while components in essential oils like lemongrass, cinnamon, citronella, rose, and peppermint were active against five tested food-spoilage fungi.[128] To destroy fungi and preserve food longer, spray produce with a mixture of 3 drops of thyme oil, 2 drops of oregano oil, and 2 drops of lemon oil in a cup of water. Rinse after fifteen minutes. Oils can be diffused in the kitchen to attack spores in the air and prevent their spread.

89. MOSQUITO REPELLANT

Mosquitos are hardy pests that have been around for millions of years. They are tough to get rid of and even tougher to avoid when outside. The females bite humans in order to use their blood to develop their fertile eggs. As they do, they inject saliva into the skin, which can cause an immune system response. The results are tiny red spots in some people or itchy, swollen red welts in others. Mosquitos can smell their prey from up to fifty meters away and are attracted to carbon dioxide, movement, chemicals in sweat, and heat. Getting bitten by a mosquito may not seem like such a big deal, but these pesky insects can carry diseases like West Nile virus, Zika virus, malaria, and yellow fever. To avoid getting bitten, many people use chemical repellent sprays or lotions on their skin. Chemical repellent paper strips worn on the body or placed in an outdoor area are used by some to avoid direct application to the skin.

Many want to avoid chemical-based repellents and are turning to natural products as alternatives. One study found that a nanoemulsion combination of 5 percent hairy basil oil, 5 percent vetiver oil, and 10 percent citronella oil was able to protect against mosquitos for 4.7 hours.[129] Other essential oils used to repel mosquitos are rosemary, peppermint, lemongrass, citronella, lavender, eucalyptus, clove, and orange. To make a body serum, combine 1 tablespoon of virgin coconut oil with 2 drops of rosemary oil, 2 drops of vetiver oil, and 5 drops of citronella oil. Smooth over the skin and reapply as needed. If mosquitos do manage to bite, dab diluted lavender on the area to soothe the skin and take out the itch.

CLEAN PATROL

90. BATHROOMS

Toilets, sinks, showers, baths, and floors in a bathroom can be a breeding ground for bacteria, viruses, and fungi if not cleaned frequently and thoroughly. Toilet seats, for example, have about fifty bacteria per square inch. That may seem like a lot, but it's really not, considering the human body houses one hundred trillion microbes. The good news is that a very small percentage of the germs encountered here are pathogenic and likely to cause illness. Gastrointestinal and foodborne viruses can last up to a week on solid surfaces and can induce diarrhea and vomiting if picked up by unsuspecting individuals. Simply flushing a toilet and then touching your mouth, nose, or eyes can transfer a pathogen from the hands and begin an infection. Other organisms can cause athlete's foot (if walking barefoot in the bathroom) or exacerbate asthma or allergies. Always wash hands after using the toilet, and make sure to sterilize toothbrushes periodically. Launder shower towels twice a week and hand towels every other day. Many products are available specifically marketed to disinfect bathrooms. They often contain ingredients that affect the respiratory system, cause skin irritation, and lead to allergies. Other ingredients are poorly biodegradable and can pollute the water systems.

HEALTH

WELL-BEING

BEAUTY

HOME

All-natural cleaners without harmful chemicals can be used with the addition of antimicrobial essential oils to eliminate bacteria, viruses, and fungi lurking on toilet seats, in the toilet bowl, and on every other surface in the bathroom. For an all-purpose cleaner, combine 2 cups of water, 2 tablespoons of castile soap, 1 tablespoon of baking soda, 30 drops of lemon essential oil, and 20 drops of rosemary essential oil. Keep in a spray bottle and shake before use. Simply spray, allow to sit on the surface for a few minutes, and wipe away. To clean inside the toilet bowl, mix 1/2 cup vinegar, 1/2 cup baking soda, and 7 drops of peppermint essential oil. Be careful, because this will fizz a lot. Pour into the bowl and scrub with a toilet brush. Other oils to choose from include lime, tea tree, eucalyptus, oregano, bergamot, cinnamon leaf, clove, citronella, and palmarosa.

91. BURNED COOKWARE

It takes only a moment's diversion to pull the cook's attention away from the sauce simmering on the stovetop or the casserole in the oven. In the span of minutes—or maybe much longer, it happens!—food can burn and get stuck on the cookware. Now there's a sticky, crusty, stuck-on mess that no amount of elbow grease will get rid of. If this happens, pour warm water in the pot or dish and gently scrape off loose bits of food using a spatula. Pour out the water and food residue. Add a few drops of lemon essential oil and let it sit for several minutes. Using a plastic scrubber, work the oil over the burned areas. They should lift out with a little effort. For a really stuck-on mess, combine the lemon oil (10 drops) with equal amounts of vinegar (1/4 cup) and baking soda (1/4 cup). Let this sit for 20 minutes, then scrub the burned areas away.

....

92. CLEANING POWER

There is a plethora of products that wipe away grime and make countertops, sinks, and windows shine. Some products cater to one job, while others are touted as all-purpose and can be used to clean just about anything. Only 7 percent of cleaning products list all their ingredients, and many contain toxic compounds that can harm your health and the environment. There are no US federal regulations for chemicals in household products, and some contain carcinogens, formaldehyde, and other highly toxic compounds known to cause reproductive, neurotoxic, and respiratory damage. These chemicals can build up in our bodies over time and trigger disease. When the product's instructions for use include wearing safety goggles and gloves and state that inhalation could be harmful or fatal, you would do well to avoid them. Even products that claim to be natural or green can still be toxic, so beware of these, too.

Simple, nontoxic cleaners can be made at home with a short list of commonly available ingredients. Perhaps the easiest all-purpose cleaner is made by combining 1 cup of warm water, 3/4 cup of apple cider vinegar, and 30 drops of essential oils. Good ones to choose from include lavender, tea tree, lemongrass, oregano, wild orange, eucalyptus, peppermint, and grapefruit. This solution will destroy germs and wash away dirt and residue on surfaces. It can be used on cutting boards, countertops (but not marble or granite), windows, sinks, microwaves, tiles, and stainless steel. Spray on and wipe off with a clean microfiber cloth.

93. FRIDGE

Refrigerators keep fresh food cool to minimize bacterial, viral, and fungal growth and maintain edibility for longer periods of time. No food is sterile, and when it gets stored in the fridge, it inevitably carries germs, which will multiply and contaminate other items. Foods host to pathogens perish more quickly, but they also run the risk of infecting consumers with harmful germs that can make them very sick. Regular fridge cleanings are recommended to prevent this from happening.

Remove food from the fridge one shelf at a time. Spray a solution of 2 cups of warm water, 1 cup of vinegar, and 15 drops of lemon essential oil over the shelf. Wipe with a clean microfiber cloth. Replace the food and move on to the next shelf. This solution will destroy germs lingering on surfaces and loosen sticky spills.

Once the fridge is clean, place a jar of 1 cup of baking soda containing 10 drops of lime, mandarin, grapefruit, or sweet orange essential oils on a shelf in the fridge to keep odors at bay. Shake the jar occasionally to release the scent. Replace the jar every four months.

94. VACUUMS

Nearly every home has a vacuum to suck up dust and dirt from floors, window coverings, and furniture. Unfortunately, most of these release some fine dust, pollen, dander, and bacteria back into the air, which can trigger asthma and allergies. Considering people spend about 90 percent of their time indoors, this chronic exposure can cause significant problems for some. Even vacuums with HEPA filters re-suspend dust and bacteria, although they are better than conventional filters. It's an aesthetic issue as well as a health issue. For those who are not prone to respiratory or allergic conditions, dust spewed back into the air can make the house smell old, dusty, musty, and just all-around unpleasant.

Before vacuuming, wipe down the outside of the vacuum to remove dust and debris. Then clean the filter pads, or change them, if disposable. Dust any accessible interior parts. Add 3 drops of any antimicrobial essential oil like lavender, tea tree, lemongrass, mandarin, manuka, oregano, rose, sage, sandalwood, peppermint, eucalyptus, bergamot, or sweet orange to the filter pad. Add another 3 drops to a cotton ball and place it in the vacuum bag or canister. When the vacuum is turned on, the essential oils will disperse through the air. Not only will they leave a pleasant aroma in the home, they will work to destroy harmful germs in the air.

HEALTH

WELL-BEING

BEAUTY

HOME

ODoR CONTROL

95. CARPETS

Carpets warm up a room, add color and texture, and provide a comfortable area for kids and pets to play. Regular vacuuming will remove surface dirt, but over time, dust and stains make their way into the fibers of the carpet and a deeper cleaning is needed. Aim to wash rugs every twelve to eighteen months. High-traffic areas, however, will require more frequent deep cleaning—every four to six months. In between deep cleanings, deodorize carpets with essential oils to remove pet, food, smoke, or any other odors that have been absorbed by the carpet fibers over time. Combine 1 cup of baking soda or borax with 20 drops of lavender essential oil in a jar and shake up. Sprinkle over the carpet, and let it sit for several hours. Vacuum up. It may take several passes to get all the baking soda out of the carpet, but the refreshing scent will prove the effort worthwhile. Orange, lime, geranium, peppermint, or any other pleasing essential oils can be used in place of, or in addition to, lavender.

96. CIGARETTE SMOKE

One of the hardest smells to eliminate in a home comes from cigarette smoke. This odor gets into everything—furniture, carpets, drapes, mattresses, floors, windows, walls, and ceilings. Even if smoking takes place only in a confined area of the house, the air filtration system will disperse the odor throughout the entire home. The odor isn't the only problem. Over 4000 chemicals are emitted in cigarette smoke, and they stain all surfaces a yellowish-brown color and leave a sticky reside.

Make sure to ventilate the house by opening windows and changing the air filters. All soft surfaces like upholstered furniture, mattresses, pillows, bedding, and carpets need to be thoroughly cleaned and deodorized. If machine washable, add 1/2 cup of apple cider vinegar and 3 drops of lavender essential oil to the washing machine to remove the smoke smell. For all other soft surfaces, after cleaning, sprinkle generously with a mixture of 1 cup baking soda and 20 drops lemongrass essential oil. Let this remain on the surface for a day, then vacuum up.

A second treatment may be necessary, depending on how deeply the odor has penetrated. Wash down walls, windows, and ceilings with a 1:1 solution of vinegar and water. Add any pleasing combination of essential oils to the solution. For a general air freshener, choose bergamot, grapefruit, or sage essential oils and add a few drops to a diffuser or spray a mixture of 1 cup of water with 10 drops of eucalyptus and rosemary essential oils into the air.

HEALTH

WELL-BEING

BEAUTY

HOME

HEALTH

WELL-BEING

BEAUTY

HOME

97. LINGERING FOOD

The aroma of baking cookies is welcome in the home, but the over-powering stench of fried fish or cabbage rolls lingering in the air is not enjoyable. While cooking, close doors to other rooms and open windows in the kitchen, if it's not too cold or hot outside. Use the ventilation fan over the stove and clean up dishes soon after the meal has ended. Remove any perishable garbage, and put it outside or in the garage. If there's room, another option is to put the smelly perishables in a bag in the freezer until garbage day.

To mask unpleasant odors, many people turn to artificial scents in candles, plug-ins, and sprays. These contain toxic chemicals that can be inhaled and cause respiratory irritation in asthmatics and those with allergies. Essential oils can be used as natural, safe alternatives to remove bad odors from the air. On the stove, simmer 2 cups of water and combine 7 to 10 drops of a combination of clove, cinnamon leaf, lemon, orange, or grapefruit essential oils. These provide a rich, fresh scent to the kitchen. If heading out for the day, place 1/2 cup of baking soda in a jar mixed with 10 drops of your favorite essential oil(s). Leave it on the counter. Foul odors will be absorbed, and the essential oils will impart a pleasing fragrance.

98. PAINT FuMES

Nothing freshens up a room like a new coat of paint. Water-based paints are most commonly used for in-home projects. These appear to be the safest, although they can still induce skin irritation on contact or vomiting if swallowed. If oil-based paints are inhaled, they can cause trouble breathing, headaches, dizziness, and nausea. When painting at home, use water-based paints, if possible. These paints have lower levels of toxic emissions and emit less odor. Always ensure adequate ventilation by keeping windows open and wear a mask to cover the mouth and nose.

Despite these measures, paint fumes will still be noticeable. Adding 80 to 100 drops of essential oils to 1 gallon of paint prior to painting will minimize the odor and, in some cases, eliminate it entirely. Peppermint is a good choice because of its strong aroma and universal appeal. Different rooms may benefit from different essential oils. If painting a bedroom, add calming oils like lavender or geranium. Fresh and spicy oils like lemon or basil would be great in the kitchen, and cypress or lemongrass are energizing oils that would favor social gatherings in the living room.

99. PETS

Pets primarily kept as working animals to herd cattle or keep mice populations in check are becoming less and less common. Now people want their pets indoors to keep them company and often give them free reign to sleep in their beds and snuggle on the furniture. Animals don't smell like humans, and they leave their noticeable scent all over the house. It may not be apparent to the pet owner, but any visitors will think they've stepped into a kennel. Aside from bathing and grooming your pet, vacuum the house regularly, wash linens and blankets, and be on the lookout for urine and other bodily substances that could be hiding in the corner of a closet or under the stairs. Stains that are not removed promptly can become difficult to eliminate.

Essential oils can banish offending pet odors and clean and refresh the home. For a general air freshener, combine 1 cup of water with 10 drops of your favorite essential oils in a spray bottle. Shake well and spray into the air all over the house. If pet urine stains are a problem, first soak up the urine with a paper towel. Wash the area with club soda and blot dry. Then spray the following mixture directly onto the stain: 1/2 cup of hydrogen peroxide, 1 teaspoon of apple cider vinegar, 1 teaspoon of baking soda (be prepared for fizzy action), and 3 drops of lemon essential oil. Allow the spray to dry on the carpet and vacuum. If any odor remains, sprinkle the area with a combination of 1/2 cup of baking soda and 5 drops of tea tree essential oil. Let this sit for a few hours and then vacuum. Other oils to use are lemongrass, lavender, rosemary, and wild orange.

100. SPORTS GEAR

Athletic clothing and equipment are subjected to sweat and body oils each time they are worn. Over a short period, this provides a breeding ground for odor-causing bacteria. These bacteria thrive and multiply, making the smells more pungent and difficult to get rid of. Fill a sink with cold water and add 1 cup of apple cider vinegar and 10 drops of tea tree oil. Allow the equipment or clothes to soak for 30 minutes. If washable, transfer them to a washing machine and wash them in cold water. Add 1/2 cup of apple cider vinegar and a few drops of any essential oil to help remove the odors and replace them with an agreeable aroma. Do not use a fabric softener. Air dry or machine dry on low heat. For equipment that can't be machine washed, simply roll them in a towel after removing them from the vinegar bath and squeeze out all the excess liquid. Then air dry in the sun, if possible.

If you don't have time for the vinegar bath but need a quick freshening, spritz equipment with a solution of 1 cup of water, 1/2 cup of witch hazel, and 300 to 350 drops of neroli, tea tree, and eucalyptus essential oils. This spray is a higher concentration than what is recommended for the skin, so use this as an equipment spray only. It will neutralize odor and kill bacteria and yeast on the equipment.

101. TRASH BINS

Spoiled food or perishables left over from meals are the main culprits in creating the stinky, rotten smell wafting from trash bins. Removing trash from the kitchen and taking it to the garage until garbage day will help reduce odors, but sometimes, they tend to stick to the trash receptacle despite being empty. Regular cleanings with soap and water will clean up any spilled liquid and bits of food stuck to the sides and bottom of the bin. Once dry, sprinkle 1 tablespoon of baking soda mixed with 5 drops of wild orange essential oil over the bottom of the bin. The odors should disappear and be replaced by a fresh orange aroma. Regularly vacuum this up and replace with a fresh batch. Adding a few drops of lavender or eucalyptus essential oil to a cotton ball and placing at the bottom of the bin, beneath the garbage bag, will also make the trash bin smell wonderful.

HEALTH

WELL-BEING

BEAUTY

HOME

NOTES

1. Higley, Connie, Pat Leatham, and Alan Higley. *Aromatherapy A-Z*. Carlsbad, California: Hay House, 1998.

2. Ibid.

3. Sturgeon, Bradley E. 2008. "Light Absorption by Various Beer Bottle Glass." Monmouth College Department of Chemistry, Monmouth, Illinois. http://www.edenfoods.com/articles/view.php?articles_id=181.

4. Higley, *Aromatherapy A-Z*.

5. Price, Shirley, and Len Price. *Aromatherapy for Health Professionals*, 3rd Ed. Philadelphia: Churchill Livingstone, 2007.

6. Asgarshirazi, Masoumeh, Mamak Shariat, and Hosein Dalili. 2015. "Comparison of the effects of pH-dependent peppermint oil and synbiotic lactol (Bacillus coagulans + Fructooligosaccharides) on childhood functional abdominal pain: a randomized placebo-controlled study." *Iran Red Crescent Medical Journal* 17 (4): e23844.

7. Kim, H. M., and S. H. Cho. 1999. "Lavender oil inhibits immediate-type allergic reaction in mice and rats." *Journal of Pharmacy and Pharmacology* 51 (2): 221–6.

8. Arthritis Foundation website, https://www.arthritis.org.

9. Wruck, C. J., A. Fragoulis, A. Gurzynski, L. O. Brandenburg, Y. W. Kan, K. Chan, J. Hassenpflug, S. Freitag-Wolf, D. Varoga, S. Lippross, and T. Pufe. 2011. "Role of oxidative stress in rheumatoid arthritis: insights from the Nrf2-knockout mice." *Annals of the Rheumatic Diseases* 70 (5): 844–50.

10. Komeh-Nkrumah, Steva A., Siddaraju M. Nanjundaiah, Rajesh Rajaiah, Hua Yu, and Kamal D. Moudgil. 2012. "Topical dermal application of essential oils attenuates the severity of adjuvant arthritis in Lewis rats." *Phytotherapy Research* 26 (1): 54–9.

11. Pattnaik, S., V. R. Subramanyam, and C. Kole. 1996. "Antibacterial and antifungal activity of ten essential oils in vitro." *Microbios* 86 (349): 237–46.

12. Frank, Mark Barton, Qing Yang, Jeanette Osban, Joseph T. Azzarello, Marcia R. Saban, Ricardo Saban, Richard A. Ashley, Jan C. Welter, Kar-Ming Fung, and Hsueh-Kung Lin. 2009. "Frankincense oil derived from Boswellia carteri induces tumor cell specific cytotoxicity." *BMC Complementary and Alternative Medicine* 9: 6.

13. Kohara, H., T. Miyauchi, Y. Suehiro, H. Ueoka, H. Takeyama, and T. Morita. 2004. "Combined modality treatment of aromatherapy, footsoak, and reflexology relieves fatigue in patients with cancer." *Journal of Palliative Medicine* 7 (6): 791–6.

14. D'Auria, F. D., M. Tecca, V. Strippoli, G. Salvatore, L. Battinelli, and G. Mazzanti. 2005. "Antifungal activity of Lavandula angustifolia essential oil against Candida albicans yeast and mycelial form." *Medical Mycology* 43 (5): 391–6.

15. Boonchild, C., and T. W. Flegel. 1982. "In vitro antifungal activity of eugenol and vanillin against Candida albicans and Cryptococcus neoformans." *Canadian Journal of Microbiology* 28 (11): 1235–41.

16. Shapiro, S., A. Meier, and B. Guggenheim. 1994. "The antimicrobial activity of essential oils and essential oil components towards oral bacteria." *Oral Microbiology and Immunology* 9: 202–8.

17. Wu, Shuhua, Krupa B. Patel, Leland J. Booth, Jordan P. Metcalf, Hsueh-Kung Lin, and Wenxin Wu. 2010. "Protective essential oil attenuates influenza virus infection: an in vitro study in MDCK cells." *BMC Complementary and Alternative Medicine* 10: 69.

18. Minami, M., M. Kita, T. Nakaya, T. Yamamoto, H. Kuriyama, and J. Imanishi. 2003. "The inhibitory effect of essential oils on herpes simplex virus type-1 replication in vitro." *Microbiology and Immunology* 47 (9): 681–4.

19. Kim, M. A., J. K. Sakong, E. J. Kim, E. H. Kim, and E. H. Kim. 2005. "Effect of aromatherapy massage for the relief of constipation in the elderly." *Taehan Kanho Hakhoe Chi* 35 (1): 56–64.

20. Gebrehiwot, Michael, Kaleab Asres, Daniel Bisrat, Avijit Mazumder, Peter Lindemann, and Franz Bucar. 2015. "Evaluation of the wound healing property of Commiphora guidottii Chiov. ex. Guid." *BMC Complementary and Alternative Medicine* 15: 282.

21. Ibid.

22. Holmes, C., V. Hopkins, C. Hensford, V. MacLaughlin, D. Wilkinson, and H. Rosenvinge. 2002. "Lavender oil as a treatment for agitated behaviour in severe dementia: a placebo controlled study." *International Journal of Geriatric Psychiatry* 17 (4): 305–8.

23. Ballard, C. G., J. T. O'Brien, K. Reichelt, and E. K. Perry. 2002. "Aromatherapy as a safe and effective treatment for the management of agitation in severe dementia: the results of a double-blind, placebo-controlled trial with Melissa." *Journal of Clinical Psychiatry* 63 (7): 553–8.

24. Kumar, Suresh, Neeru Vasudeva, and Sunil Sharma. 2012. "GC-MS analysis and screening of antidiabetic, antioxidant and hypolipidemic potential

of Cinnamomum tamala oil in streptozotocin induced diabetes mellitus in rats." *Cardiovascular Diabetology* 11: 95.

25. Boukhris, Maher, Mohamed Bouaziz, Ines Feki, Hedya Jemai, Abdelfattah El Feki, and Sami Sayadi. 2012. "Hypoglycemic and antioxidant effects of leaf essential oil of Pelargonium graveolens L'Hér. in alloxan induced diabetic rats." *Lipids in Health and Disease* 11: 81.

26. Dorman, H. J., and S. G. Deans. 2000. "Antimicrobial agents from plants: antibacterial activity of plant volatile oils." *Journal of Applied Microbiology* 88 (2): 308–16.

27. Scandorieiro, Sara, Larissa C. de Camargo, Cesar A. Lancheros, Sueli F. Yamada-Ogatta, Celso V. Nakamura, Admilton G. de Oliveira, Célia G. Andrade, Nelson Duran, Gerson Nakazato, and Renata K. Kobayashi. 2016. "Synergistic and additive effect of oregano essential oil and biological silver nanoparticles against multidrug-resistant bacterial strains." *Frontiers in Microbiology* 7: 760.

28. Aridoğan, B. C., H. Baydar, S. Kaya, M. Demirci, D. Ozbaşar, and E. Mumcu. 2002. "Antimicrobial activity and chemical composition of some essential oils." *Archives of Pharmacal Research* 25 (6): 860–4.

29. Meamarbashi, Abbas, and Ali Rajabi. 2013. "The effects of peppermint on exercise performance." *Journal of the International Society of Sports Nutrition* 10: 15.

30. Singh, Surender, and D. K. Majumdar. 1995. "Anti-inflammatory and antipyretic activities of ocimum sanctum fixed oil." *International Journal of Pharmacognosy* 33 (4): 288–92.

31. Feng, J., and J. M. Lipton. 1987. "Eugenol: antipyretic activity in rabbits." *Neuropharmacology* 26 (12): 1775–8.

32. Queiroz, João Carlos, Ângelo R. Antoniolli, Lucindo J. Quintans-Júnior, Renan G. Brito, Rosana S. S. Barreto, Emmanoel V. Costa, Thanany B. da Silva, Ana Paula Nascimento Prata, Waldecy de Lucca Júnior, Jackson R. Almeida, Julianeli T. Lima, and Jullyana Quintans. 2014. "Evaluation of the anti-inflammatory and antinociceptive effects of the essential oil from leaves of Xylopia laevigata in experimental models." *Scientific World Journal* 2014: 816450.

33. Nascimento, Simone S., Adriano A. Araújo, Renan G. Brito, Mairim R. Serafini, Paula P. Menezes, Josimari M. DeSantana, Waldecy de Lucca Júnior, Pericles B. Alves, Arie F. Blank, Rita C. Oliveira, Aldeidia P. Oliveira, Ricardo L. Albuquerque-Júnior, Jackson R. Almeida, and Lucindo J. Quintans-Júnior. 2014. "Cyclodextrin-complexed Ocimum basilicum leaves essential oil increases Fos protein expression in the central nervous system and produces

an antihyperalgesic effect in animal models for fibromyalgia." *International Journal of Molecular Sciences* 16 (1): 547–63.

34. Aloisi, A. M., I. Ceccarelli, F. Masi, and A. Scaramuzzino. 2002. "Effects of the essential oil from citrus lemon in male and female rats exposed to a persistent painful stimulation." *Behavioral Brain Research* 136 (1): 127–35.

35. Wu K. L, C. K. Rayner, S. K. Chuah, C. S. Changchien, S. N. Lu, Y. C. Chiu, K. W. Chiu, and C. M. Lee. 2008. "Effects of ginger on gastric emptying and motility in healthy humans." *European Journal of Gastroenterology and Hepatology* 20 (5): 436–40.

36. Rocha Caldas, Germana Freire, Alisson Rodrigo da Silva Oliveira, Alice Valença Araújo, Dafne Carolina Alves Quixabeira, Jacinto da Costa Silva-Neto, João Henrique Costa-Silva, Irwin Rose Alencar de Menezes, Fabiano Ferreira, Ana Cristina Lima Leite, José Galberto Martins da Costa, and Almir Gonçalves Wanderley. 2014. "Gastroprotective and ulcer healing effects of essential oil of Hyptis martiusii Benth. (Lamiaceae)." *PLOS One* 9 (1): e84400.

37. Guesmi, Fatma, Manel Ben Ali, Taha Barkaoui, Wiem Tahri, Mondher Mejri, Mossadok Ben-Attia, Houda Bellamine, and Ahmed Landoulsi. 2014. "Effects of Thymus hirtus sp. algeriensis Boiss. et Reut. (Lamiaceae) essential oil on healing gastric ulcers according to sex." *Lipids in Health and Disease* 13: 138.

38. Imai, H., K. Osawa, H. Yasuda, H. Hamashima, T. Arai, and M. Sasatsu. 2001. "Inhibition by the essential oils of peppermint and spearmint of the growth of pathogenic bacteria." *Microbios* 106 (Suppl 1): 31–9.

39. Rodrigues, Ítalo Sarto Carvalho, Vinícius Nascimento Tavares, Sérgio Luís da Silva Pereira, and Flávio Nogueira da Costa. 2009. "Antiplaque and anti-gingivitis effect of Lippia sidoides: a double-blind clinical study in humans." *Journal of Applied Oral Science* 17 (5): 404–7.

40. Göbel, H., J. Fresenius, A. Heinze, M. Dworschak, and D. Soyka. 1996. "Effectiveness of Oleum menthae piperitae and paracetamol in therapy of headache of the tension type." *Der Nervenarzt* 67 (8): 672–81.

41. Sasannejad, P., M. Saeedi, A. Shoeibi, A. Gorji, M. Abbasi, M. Foroughipour. 2012. "Lavender essential oil in the treatment of migraine headache: a placebo-controlled clinical trial." *European Neurology* 67 (5): 288–91.

42. Ahmad, Shafeeque, and Zafarul H. Beg. 2013. "Elucidation of mechanisms of actions of thymoquinone-enriched methanolic and volatile oil extracts from Nigella sativa against cardiovascular risk parameters in experimental hyperlipidemia." *Lipids in Health and Disease* 12: 86.

43. Shalaby, Mostafa Abbas, and Ashraf Abd-Elkhalik Hammouda. 2014. "Analgesic, anti-inflammatory and anti-hyperlipidemic activities of Commiphora molmol extract (Myrrh)." *Journal of Intercultural Ethnopharmacology* 3 (2): 56–62.

44. Cha, J. H., S. H. Lee, and Y. S. Yoo. 2010. "Effects of aromatherapy on changes in the autonomic nervous system, aortic pulse wave velocity and aortic augmentation index in patients with essential hypertension." *Journal of Korean Academy of Nursing* 40 (5): 705–13.

45. Hwang, J. H. 2006. "The effects of the inhalation method using essential oils on blood pressure and stress responses of clients with essential hypertension." *Taehan Kanho Hakhoe Chi* 36 (7): 1123–34.

46. Komori, T., R. Fujiwara, M. Tanida, J. Nomura, and M. M. Yokoyama. 1995. "Effects of citrus fragrance on immune function and depressive states." *Neuroimmunomodulation* 2 (3): 174–80.

47. Baratta, M. Tiziana, H. J. Damien Dorman, Stanley G. Deans, Daniela M. Biondi, and Giuseppe Ruberto. 1998. "Chemical composition, antimicrobial and antioxidative activity of laurel, sage, rosemary, oregano and coriander essential oils." *Journal of Essential Oil Research* 10 (6): 618–27.

48. Kumar, "GC-MS analysis and screening of antidiabetic, antioxidant and hypolipidemic potential of Cinnamomum tamala oil in streptozotocin induced diabetes mellitus in rats."

49. Boukhris, "Hypoglycemic and antioxidant effects of leaf essential oil of Pelargonium graveolens L'Hér. in alloxan induced diabetic rats."

50. Queiroz, "Evaluation of the anti-inflammatory and antinociceptive effects of the essential oil from leaves of Xylopia laevigata in experimental models."

51. Pinheiro, Mariana Martins, Ana B. Miltojević, Niko S. Radulović, Ikarastika Rahayu Abdul-Wahab, Fabio Boylan, and Patrícia Dias Fernandes. 2015. "Anti-inflammatory activity of Choisya ternata Kunth essential oil, ternanthranin, and its two synthetic analogs (methyl and propyl N-methylanthranilates)." *PLOS One* 10 (3): e0121063.

52. Shalaby, "Analgesic, anti-inflammatory and anti-hyperlipidemic activities of *Commiphora molmol* extract (Myrrh)."

53. Komeh-Nkrumah, "Topical dermal application of essential oils attenuates the severity of adjuvant arthritis in Lewis rats."

54. Nascimento, "Cyclodextrin-complexed Ocimum basilicum leaves essential oil increases Fos protein expression in the central nervous system and produces an antihyperalgesic effect in animal models for fibromyalgia."

55. Aloisi, "Effects of the essential oil from citrus lemon in male and female rats exposed to a persistent painful stimulation."

56. Keshavarz Afshar, M., Z. Behboodi Moghadam, Z. Taghizadeh, R. Bekhradi, A. Montazeri, and P. Mokhtari. 2015. "Lavender fragrance essential oil and the quality of sleep in postpartum women." *Iran Red Crescent Medical Journal* 17 (4): 25880.

57. Diego, M. A., N. A. Jones, T. Field, M. Hernandez-Reif, S. Schanberg, C. Kuhn, V. McAdam, R. Galamaga, and M. Galamaga. 1998. "Aromatherapy positively affects mood, EEG patterns of alertness and math computations." *The International Journal of Neuroscience* 96 (3–4): 217–24.

58. Ali, Babar, Naser Ali Al-Wabel, Saiba Shams, Aftab Ahamad, Shah Alam Khan, and Firoz Anwar. 2015. "Essential oils used in aromatherapy: a systemic review." *Asian Pacific Journal of Tropical Biomedicine* 5 (8): 601–11.

59. Cash, Brooks D., Michael S. Epstein, and Syed M. Shah. 2016. "A novel delivery system of peppermint oil is an effective therapy for irritable bowel syndrome symptoms." *Digestive Diseases and Sciences* 61: 560–71.

60. Ro, Y. J., H. C. Ha, C. G. Kim, and H. A. Yeom. 2002. "The effects of aromatherapy on pruritus in patients undergoing hemodialysis." *Dermatology Nursing* 14 (4): 231–4, 237–8, 256.

61. Diego, "Aromatherapy positively affects mood, EEG patterns of alertness and math computations."

62. Ali, "Essential oils used in aromatherapy: a systemic review."

63. Diego, "Aromatherapy positively affects mood, EEG patterns of alertness and math computations."

64. Barker, Stephen C., and Phillip M. Altman. 2010. "A randomised, assessor blind, parallel group comparative efficacy trial of three products for the treatment of head lice in children—melaleuca oil and lavender oil, pyrethrins and piperonyl butoxide, and a 'suffocation' product." *BMC Dermatology* 10: 6.

65. Ibid.

66. De Oliveira, T. L., M. das Graças Cardoso, R. de Araújo Soares, E. M. Ramos, R. H. Piccoli, and V. M. Tebaldi. 2013. "Inhibitory activity of Syzygium aromaticum and Cymbopogon citratus (DC.) Stapf. essential oils against Listeria monocytogenes inoculated in bovine ground meat." *Brazilian Journal of Microbiology* 44 (2): 357–65.

67. Mossa, Abdel-Tawab H., Amel A. Refaie, Amal Ramadan, and Jalloul Bouajila. 2013. "Amelioration of prallethrin-induced oxidative stress and hepatotoxicity in rat by the administration of Origanum majorana essential oil." *BioMed Research International* 2013: 859085.

68. Ou, M. C., T. F. Hsu, A. C. Lai, Y. T. Lin, and C. C. Lin. 2012. "Pain relief assessment by aromatic essential oil massage on outpatients with primary dysmenorrhea: a randomized, double-blind clinical trial." *Journal of Obstetrics and Gynaecology Research* 38 (5): 817–22.

69. Han, S. H., M. H. Hur, J. Buckle, J. Choi, and M. S. Lee. 2006. "Effect of aromatherapy on symptoms of dysmenorrhea in college students: a randomized placebo-controlled clinical trial." *Journal of Alternative and Complementary Medicine* 12 (6): 535–41.

70. Tate, S. 1997. "Peppermint oil: a treatment for postoperative nausea." *Journal of Advanced Nursing* 26 (3): 543–9.

71. Davies, S. J., L. M. Harding, and A. P. Baranowski. 2002. "A novel treatment of postherpetic neuralgia using peppermint oil." *Clinical Journal of Pain* 18 (3): 200–2.

72. Li, L. 2010. "The effect of Neuragen PN on neuropathic pain: a randomized, double blind, placebo controlled clinical trial." *BMC Complementary and Alternative Medicine* 10: 22.

73. D'Auria, "Antifungal activity of Lavandula angustifolia essential oil against Candida albicans yeast and mycelial form."

74. Labib, Gihan S., and Hibah Aldawsari. 2015. "Innovation of natural essential oil-loaded Orabase for local treatment of oral candidiasis." *Drug Design, Development and Therapy* 9: 3349–59.

75. Ni, Xiao, Mahmoud M. Suhail, Qing Yang, Amy Cao, Kar-Ming Fung, Russell G. Postier, Cole Woolley, Gary Young, Jingzhe Zhang, and Hsueh-Kung Lin. 2012. "Frankincense essential oil prepared from hydrodistillation of Boswellia sacra gum resins induces human pancreatic cancer cell death in cultures and in a xenograft murine model." *BMC Complementary and Alternative Medicine* 12: 253.

76. Dale, A., and S. Cornwell. 1994. "The role of lavender oil in relieving perineal discomfort following childbirth: a blind randomized clinical trial." *Journal of Advanced Nursing* 19 (1): 89–96.

77. Pimentel, Suzana Peres, Guilherme Emerson Barrella, Renato Corrêa Casarin, Fabiano Ribeiro Cirano, Márcio Zaffalon Casati, Mary Ann Foglio, Glyn Mara Figueira, and Fernanda Vieira Ribeiro. 2012. "Protective effect of topical Cordia verbenacea in a rat periodontitis model: immune-inflammatory, antibacterial and morphometric assays." *BMC Complementary and Alternative Medicine* 12: 224.

78. Suresh, P., V. K. Ingle, and V. Vijayalakshmi. 1992. "Antibacterial activity of eugenol in comparison with other antibiotics." *Journal of Food Science and Technology* 29: 256–7.

79. Pinheiro, "Anti-inflammatory activity of Choisya ternata Kunth essential oil, ternanthranin, and its two synthetic analogs (methyl and propyl N-methylanthranilates)."

80. Shalaby, "Analgesic, anti-inflammatory and anti-hyperlipidemic activities of *Commiphora molmol* extract (Myrrh)."

81. Komeh-Nkrumah, "Topical dermal application of essential oils attenuates the severity of adjuvant arthritis in Lewis rats."

82. Nenoff, P., U. F. Haustein, and W. Brandt. 1996. "Antifungal activity of the essential oil of Melaleuca alternifolia (tea tree oil) against pathogenic fungi

in vitro." *Skin Pharmacology* 9 (6): 388–94.

83. Thomas, Jackson, Christine F. Carson, Greg M. Peterson, Shelley F. Walton, Kate A. Hammer, Mark Naunton, Rachel C. Davey, Tim Spelman, Pascale Dettwiller, Greg Kyle, Gabrielle M. Cooper, and Kavya E. Baby. 2016. "Therapeutic potential of tea tree oil for scabies." *The American Journal of Tropical Medicine and Hygiene* 94 (2): 258–66.

84. Karimzadeh, Fariba, Mahmoud Hosseini, Diana Mangeng, Hassan Alavi, Gholam Reza Hassanzadeh, Mohamad Bayat, Maryam Jafarian, Hadi Kazemi, and Ali Gorji. 2012. "Anticonvulsant and neuroprotective effects of *Pimpinella anisum* in rat brain." *BMC Complementary and Alternative Medicine* 12: 76.

85. Rose, J. E., and F. M. Behm. 1994. "Inhalation of vapor from black pepper extract reduces smoking withdrawal symptoms." *Drug and Alcohol Dependence* 34 (3): 225–9.

86. Carson, C. F., B. D. Cookson, H. D. Farrelly, and T. V. Riley. 1995. "Susceptibility of methicillin-resistant Staphylococcus aureus to the essential oil of Melaleuca alternifolia." *Journal of Antimicrobial Chemotherapy* 35 (3): 421–4.

87. Dryden, M. S., S. Dailly, and M. Crouch. 2004. "A randomized, controlled trial of tea tree topical preparations versus a standard topical regimen for the clearance of MRSA colonization." *Journal of Hospital Infection* 56 (4): 283–6.

88. Edwards-Jones, V., R. Buck, S. G. Shawcross, M. M. Dawson, and K. Dunn. 2004. "The effect of essential oils on methicillin-resistant Staphylococcus aureus using a dressing model." *Burns* 30 (8): 772–7.

89. Nelson, R. R. S. 1997. "In-vitro activities of five plant essential oils against methicillin-resistant Staphylococcus aureus and vancomycin-resistant Enterococcus faecium." *Journal of Antimicrobial Chemotherapy* 40 (2): 305–6.

90. Aridoğan, "Antimicrobial activity and chemical composition of some essential oils."

91. Nenoff, "Antifungal activity of the essential oil of Melaleuca alternifolia (tea tree oil) against pathogenic fungi in vitro."

92. Pietrella, Donatella, Letizia Angiolella, Elisabetta Vavala, Anna Rachini, Francesca Mondello, Rino Ragno, Francesco Bistoni, and Anna Vecchiarelli. 2011. "Beneficial effect of Mentha suaveolens essential oil in the treatment of vaginal candidiasis assessed by real-time monitoring of infection." *BMC Complementary and Alternative Medicine* 11: 18.

93. D'Auria, "Antifungal activity of Lavandula angustifolia essential oil against Candida albicans yeast and mycelial form."

94. De Campos Rasteiro, Vanessa Maria, Anna Carolina Borges Pereira da Costa, Cássia Fernandes Araújo, Patrícia Pimentel de Barros, Rodnei Dennis Rossoni, Ana Lia Anbinder, Antonio Olavo Cardoso Jorge, and Juliana Campos Junqueira. 2014. "Essential oil of Melaleuca alternifolia for the treatment of oral candidiasis induced in an immunosuppressed mouse model." *BMC Complementary and Alternative Medicine* 14: 489.

95. Batubara, Irmanida, Irma H. Suparto, Siti Sa'diah, Ryunosuke Matsuoka, and Tohru Mitsunaga. 2015. "Effects of inhaled citronella oil and related compounds on rat body weight and brown adipose tissue sympathetic nerve." *Nutrients* 7 (3): 1859–70.

96. Hursel, R., and M. S. Westerterp-Plantenga. 2010. "Thermogenic ingredients and body weight regulation." *International Journal of Obesity* 34 (4): 659–69.

97. Warnke, P. H., E. Sherry, P. A. Russo, Y. Açil, J. Wiltfang, S. Sivananthan, M. Sprengel, J. C. Roldàn, S. Schubert, J. P. Bredee, and I. N. Springer. 2006. "Antibacterial essential oils in malodorous cancer patients: clinical observations in 30 patients." *Phytomedicine* 13 (7): 463–7.

98. Higley, *Aromatherapy A-Z*.

99. Ibid.

100. Costa, Celso A. R. A., Thaís C. Cury, Bruna O. Cassettari, Regina K. Takahira, Jorge C. Flório, and Mirtes Costa. 2013. "Citrus aurantium L. essential oil exhibits anxiolytic-like activity mediated by 5-HT$_{1A}$-receptors and reduces cholesterol after repeated oral treatment." *BMC Complementary and Alternative Medicine* 13: 42.

101. Itai, T., H. Amayasu, M. Kuribayashi, N. Kawamura, M. Okada, A. Momose, T. Tateyama, K. Narumi, W. Uematsu, and S. Kaneko. 2000. "Psychological effects of aromatherapy on chronic hemodialysis patients." *Psychiatry and Clinical Neurosciences* 54 (4): 393–7.

102. Diego, "Aromatherapy positively affects mood, EEG patterns of alertness and math computations."

103. Wilkinson, S., J. Aldridge, I. Salmon, E. Cain, and B. Wilson. 1999. "An evaluation of aromatherapy massage in palliative care." *Palliative Medicine* 13 (5): 409–17.

104. Grady, Cheryl L., Mellanie V. Springer, Donaya Hongwanishkul, Anthony R. McIntosh, and Gordon Winocur. 2006. "Age-related changes in brain activity across the adult lifespan." *Journal of Cognitive Neuroscience* 18 (2): 227–41.

105. Komori, "Effects of citrus fragrance on immune function and depressive states."

106. Itai, "Psychological effects of aromatherapy on chronic hemodialysis patients."

107. Diego, "Aromatherapy positively affects mood, EEG patterns of alertness and math computations."

108. Matsumoto, Tamaki, Hiroyuki Asakura, and Tatsuya Hayashi. 2014. "Effects of olfactory stimulation from the fragrance of the Japanese citrus fruit yuzu (Citrus junos Sieb. ex Tanaka) on mood states and salivary chromogranin A as an endocrinologic stress marker." *Journal of Alternative and Complementary Medicine* 20 (6): 500–6.

109. Motomura, N., A. Sakurai, and Y. Yotsuya. 2001. "Reduction of mental stress with lavender odorant." *Perceptual and Motor Skills* 93 (3): 713–8.

110. Mesfin, Miraf, Kaleab Asres, and Workineh Shibeshi. 2014. "Evaluation of anxiolytic activity of the essential oil of the aerial part of Foeniculum vulgare Miller in mice." *BMC Complementary and Alternative Medicine* 14: 310.

111. Fu, Y., Y. Zu, L. Chen, T. Efferth, H. Liang, Z. Liu, W. Liu. 2007. "Investigation of antibacterial activity of rosemary essential oil against Propionibacterium acnes with atomic force microscopy." *Planta Medica* 73 (12): 1275–80.

112. Satchell, A. C., A. Saurajen, C. Bell, and R. S. Barnetson. 2002. "Treatment of dandruff with 5% tea tree oil shampoo." *Journal of the American Academy of Dermatology* 47 (6): 852–5.

113. Nenoff, "Antifungal activity of the essential oil of Melaleuca alternifolia (tea tree oil) against pathogenic fungi in vitro."

114. Pimentel, "Protective effect of topical Cordia verbenacea in a rat periodontitis model."

115. D'Auria, "Antifungal activity of Lavandula angustifolia essential oil against Candida albicans yeast and mycelial form."

116. Labib, "Innovation of natural essential oil-loaded Orabase for local treatment of oral candidiasis."

117. Hay, I. C., M. Jamieson, and A. D. Ormerod. 1998. "Randomized trial of aromatherapy: successful treatment for alopecia areata." *Archives of Dermatology* 134 (11): 1349–52.

118. Lee, Boo Hyeong, Jae Soon Lee, and Young Chul Kim. 2016. "Hair growth-promoting effects of lavender oil in C57BL/6 mice." *Toxicological Research* 32 (2): 103–8.

119. D'Auria, "Antifungal activity of Lavandula angustifolia essential oil against Candida albicans yeast and mycelial form."

120. Nenoff, "Antifungal activity of the essential oil of Melaleuca alternifolia (tea tree oil) against pathogenic fungi in vitro."

121. Zhang, Hong, Xia Ran, Chang-Ling Hu, Lu-Ping Qin, Ying Lu, and Cheng Peng. 2012. "Therapeutic effects of liposome-enveloped *Ligusticum chuanxiong* essential oil on hypertrophic scars in the rabbit ear model." *PLOS One* 7 (2): e31157.

122. Kaur, Chanchal Deep, and Swarnlata Saraf. 2010. "In vitro sun protection factor determination of herbal oils used in cosmetics." *Pharmacognosy Research* 2 (1): 22–5.

123. Ibid.

124. Shapiro, "The antimicrobial activity of essential oils and essential oil components towards oral bacteria."

125. Deans, S. G., and G. Ritchie. 1987. "Antibacterial properties of plant essential oils." *International Journal of Food Microbiology* 5 (2): 165–80.

126. Stavropoulou, Andriana, Kostas Loulakakis, Naresh Magan, and Nikos Tzortzakis. 2014. "*Origanum dictamnus* oil vapour suppresses the development of grey mould in eggplant fruit *in vitro*." *BioMed Research International* 2014: 1–11.

127. Connor, D. E., and L. R. Beuchat. 1984. "Effects of essential oils from plants on growth of food spoilage yeasts." *Journal of Food Science* 49: 429–34.

128. Moleyar, V., and P. Narasimham. 1986. "Antifungal activity of some essential oil components." *Food Microbiology* 3 (4): 331–6.

129. Nuchuchua, Onanong, Usawadee Sakulku, Napaporn Uawongyart, Satit Puttipipatkhachorn, Apinan Soottitantawat, and Uracha Ruktanonchai. 2009. "In vitro characterization and mosquito (Aedes aegypti) repellent activity of essential-oils-loaded nanoemulsions." *AAPS PharmSciTech* 10 (4): 1234–42.

ABOUT THE AUTHOR

SUSAN BRANSON earned an undergraduate degree in biology from St. Francis Xavier University, then a MSc in toxicology from the University of Ottawa. From there, she worked in research: in the field, in the lab, as a writer, and as an administrator. She took time off and stayed at home after her second child was born. In addition to being a stay-at-home mom, she also took violin lessons, photography courses, earned a diploma in writing, and ultimately became a holistic nutritional consultant. Susan is a member of CSNN's Alumni Association, Canada's leading holistic nutrition school.

ABOUT FAMILIUS

VISIT OUR WEBSITE: WWW.FAMILIUS.COM
JOIN OUR FAMILY

There are lots of ways to connect with us! Subscribe to our news-letters at www.familius.com to receive uplifting daily inspiration, essays from our Pater Familius, a free ebook every month, and the first word on special discounts and Familius news.

GET BULK DISCOUNTS

If you feel a few friends and family might benefit from what you've read, let us know and we'll be happy to provide you with quantity discounts. Simply email us at orders@familius.com.

CONNECT

Facebook: www.facebook.com/paterfamilius
Twitter: @familiustalk, @paterfamilius1
Pinterest: www.pinterest.com/familius
Instagram: @familiustalk

FAMILIUS

THE MOST IMPORTANT WORK YOU
EVER DO WILL BE WITHIN THE
WALLS OF YOUR OWN HOME.

CPSIA information can be obtained
at www.ICGtesting.com
Printed in the USA
FSOW01n1458061017
39472FS

9 781945 547164